Understanding Your Teenager's Depression

ISSUES, INSIGHTS AND PRACTICAL
GUIDANCE FOR PARENTS

Other books by Kathleen McCoy, Ph.D.

GROWING AND CHANGING: A HANDBOOK FOR PRETEENS
(with Charles Wibbelsman, M.D.)

THE SECRETS OF MY LIFE: A GIRL'S SELF-DISCOVERY JOURNAL

THE TEENAGE BODY BOOK
(with Charles Wibbelsman, M.D.)

LIFE HAPPENS
(with Charles Wibbelsman, M.D.)

CRISIS-PROOF YOUR TEENAGER

CHANGES AND CHOICES

THE TEENAGE BODY BOOK GUIDE TO DATING

THE TEENAGE BODY BOOK GUIDE TO SEXUALITY

THE TEENAGE SURVIVAL GUIDE

Most Perigee Books are available at special quantity discounts for bulk purchases for sales promotions, premiums, fund-raising, or educational use. Special books, or book excerpts, can also be created to fit specific needs.

For details, write: Special Markets, The Berkley Publishing Group, 375 Hudson Street, New York, New York 10014.

Understanding Your Teenager's Depression

ISSUES, INSIGHTS AND PRACTICAL GUIDANCE FOR PARENTS

KATHLEEN MCCOY, PH.D.

With a Foreword by
RICHARD G. MACKENZIE, M.D.
Director of the Adolescent Medicine Division
of Children's Hospital, Los Angeles

Previously published as
Coping with Teenage Depression

A PERIGEE BOOK

THE BERKLEY PUBLISHING GROUP
Published by the Penguin Group
Penguin Group (USA) Inc.
375 Hudson Street, New York, New York 10014, USA
Penguin Group (Canada), 90 Eglinton Avenue East, Suite 700, Toronto, Ontario M4P 2Y3, Canada
(a division of Pearson Penguin Canada Inc.)
Penguin Books Ltd., 80 Strand, London WC2R 0RL, England
Penguin Group Ireland, 25 St. Stephen's Green, Dublin 2, Ireland (a division of Penguin Books Ltd.)
Penguin Group (Australia), 250 Camberwell Road, Camberwell, Victoria 3124, Australia
(a division of Pearson Australia Group Pty. Ltd.)
Penguin Books India Pvt. Ltd., 11 Community Centre, Panchsheel Park, New Delhi—110 017, India
Penguin Group (NZ), Cnr. Airborne and Rosedale Roads, Albany, Auckland 1310, New Zealand
(a division of Pearson New Zealand Ltd.)
Penguin Books (South Africa) (Pty.) Ltd., 24 Sturdee Avenue, Rosebank, Johannesburg 2196,
South Africa

Penguin Books Ltd., Registered Offices: 80 Strand, London WC2R 0RL, England

The publisher does not have any control over and does not assume any responsibility for author or third-party websites or their content.

Copyright © 1994, 2005 by Kathleen McCoy
Cover art and design by Charles Björklund
Cover photo by Superstock

PRINTING HISTORY
Revised Perigee trade paperback edition / October 2005

PERIGEE is a registered trademark of Penguin Group (USA) Inc.
The "P" design is a trademark belonging to Penguin Group (USA) Inc.

The original Perigee trade paperback was cataloged by the Library of Congress as follows

McCoy, Kathy.
    Understanding your teenager's depression : issues, insights, and practical guidance for parents / by Kathleen McCoy; with a foreword by Richard G. MacKenzie.
    p. cm.
    Rev. ed. of: Coping with teenage depression, 1982.
    ISBN 0-399-51856-8
    1. Depression in adolescence.   I. McCoy, Kathy. Coping with teenage depression.   II. Title.
RJ506.D4M32   1994   93-45042 CIP
616.85'27'00835—dc20

PRINTED IN THE UNITED STATES OF AMERICA

10 9 8 7 6 5 4 3 2 1

In loving memory of Aunt Molly (Elizabeth C. McCoy) 1917–2004 . . . who gave me inspiration and hope in my teens and a lifetime of very special joy.

Contents

Acknowledgments

Special thanks to . . .

. . . Tai, who started it all, giving me painful and personal insights into the problems and challenges that teenage depression can bring to a family.

. . . Susan Ann Protter, an extraordinary literary agent, for originating the idea for this book many years ago and for her initiative and supportiveness in helping this update to happen.

. . . John Duff, the publisher and Adrienne Schultz, the editor, of this update, for their enthusiasm and support in giving this book a whole new life.

. . . All of the physicians, mental health professionals and educators whose insights and special knowledge have added so much to this book. I am particularly grateful to my dear friend and frequent collaborator Charles Wibbelsman, M.D., and to my equally dear friends Mary Breiner, M.A., MFT, and Patricia Hill. I also particularly appreciate the support of my colleagues Joyce Moore, LCSW, Stella Natelli, Leslie To, Ph.D., Kary To, Ph.D., Elaine Kindle, Ph.D., Caren Caty, Ph.D., Diane Smoot, Ph.D., Eve Seigel, M.A., MFT, Linda Gilbert, M.A., MFT, Elizabeth Canfield, Michael Obarski, Ph.D. and Michael Scavio, Ph.D.

. . . Nora Valdiviezo, my supervisor at UCLA, for her warm encouragement and support.

. . . My husband, Bob Stover, for his love and belief in me, for his unfailing patience and support during the long nights and weekends of work on this book . . . and so many others over the past thirty years of our life together.

. . . Friends and family, who contributed so much in many ways: Mike McCoy, M.D., Tai McCoy, RN, Nicky Mareld, Lawrence Mayer, M.D., Graciela Mayer, RN, Melody Mayer, Eric Mayer, Ryan Grady, Kelly Grady, Caron Roudebush, Jack Hill, Tim Schellhardt, Jeanne Yagi, Sister Rita

McCormack, Sister Ramona Bascom, Mariana and Dorothy Dusa, Diana Browne, Alicia Viramontes, Annette Sula-Goff and Jennifer Rourke.

. . . All of the teenagers and parents who took the risk of sharing their feelings and their lives with me. Their names have been changed to protect their privacy, but the people and their stories are real.

Foreword

by Dr. Richard MacKenzie

There is no use for a teenager in American society today. There was a time when a family was valued by society for the number of children it had. Children were assets, assuring the continuity of the family line. When teenagers, they actively participated in maintaining the family through assuming responsibility for a number of tasks in the home, farm, or community. They contributed to the identity of the family. They felt needed and part of the community. Parents would "showcase" their children and teenagers wherever the opportunity arose—at church, picnics, community fairs. They, in general, were proud, and the children were proud!

Teenagers felt needed and built their concept of self around this. They established their future goals, explored their fantasies, and chose their friends within the framework of this identity. Schooling was a means to this end and was, for all practical purposes, a finite experience—finite in the sense that there was a beginning, a middle, and an end; finite in the sense that goals were clear, generally centered around the three R's; finite in the sense that the time commitment was clear and the number of years of involvement, practical. Within a dozen years of concentrated schooling the world was at their feet! The dreams of wealth, respect, power, travel, security, and excitement were the fuel which helped teenagers to value the years of preparation, for one day the world would be theirs!

Today's teenagers are not without their dreams and then fantasies, but somehow they do not seem as attainable. The journey is longer. The educational route now takes decades—high school, college, graduate school—and even then there are many uncertainties. And along the way there is little use for young people, for they are in preparation. They are being molded, without permanent shape. They are not seen for who they are, but for what they can be. And yet they are not that—they are what they are. And who they are is the identity of teenagers today—confronted with the ambiguity of education, the dissolution of family, the hostile commercialism of society, and the insecurity of relationships. And this identity is fragile—threatened by fears of rejection, feelings of failure, and of being different. Panicked by a sense of isolation, teenagers make a commitment to lifestyle, to friends, to sports, to gangs, to music, to fashion. The adult confrontation promotes the isolation, the separateness, the differences, and the "you don't understand me" attitude.

Depression, as Kathleen McCoy points out, is a common concomitant to this struggle, and it is often aggravated by the very things that we think should relieve it. Being with friends may only heighten the fear of eventual rejection. Participation in sports may in the teenager's mind only spell impending failure to live up to the expectations of parents, coaches, teachers, and friends.

The paradox becomes clear—by doing, you undo: undoing in the sense that the teenager now risks losing what identity he or she has attained. With the undoing, the outward spiral of growth and exploration turns inward on itself and involutes. The depressive symptoms begin to manifest themselves. And, like many of the teenagers' messages, they are not direct. It is this indirectness which catches us off guard, both as professionals and as parents trying to help. We fail to recognize, for example, the significance of psychosomatic symptoms, school failure, drug abuse, changed eating patterns, loss of interest in pastimes or sports. That adolescent depression is a great mimicker needs to be underlined in red ink. It can fool even the most astute of professionals and parents, giving rise to the disregard of or the minimizing of complaints. When it is finally recognized, parents often feel a sense of failure and guilt which may immobilize them into a state of inaction. Dr. McCoy, having talked with teenagers, parents, and professionals, has brought together perceptions from all sides of the issue. These insights provide parents with the red ink with which they need to highlight their own teenagers' behavior. The early identification and the use of appropriate remedies within the family—or through professional help—lessens the pain to all and redirects the spiral of adolescent growth outward to excitement and new experience.

Richard G. MacKenzie, M.D., Director
Division of Adolescent Medicine
Children's Hospitals of Los Angeles

Assistant Professor of Pediatrics & Medicine
Departments of Pediatrics & Medicine
University of Southern California School of Medicine

Teenage Depression

An Introduction

Britney Caldwell was angry, oppositional and just plain ornery. She avoided family activities, didn't want to be seen with her parents, holed up in her room listening to music and, on the rare occasions when she did speak, said she hated her new school and didn't have any friends. Her parents thought that she was just hitting a rough spot in adolescence as she started her freshman year of high school. They tried to be sensitive, approachable, and supportive even as they dealt with their own frustration as their formerly sweet daughter became a surly, withdrawn stranger.

It wasn't until a teacher and school counselor called them, reporting that Britney was getting into fights at school and had been frequently truant during the past few weeks that the Caldwells began to realize that something out of the ordinary was going on with their daughter. The school counselor told them that she thought Britney was depressed. Her parents were shocked. Britney hadn't been *acting* depressed—or had she?

Such bewilderment is not unusual. A recent *Los Angeles Times* report recounted the story of the October 2004 suicide of fifteen-year-old Velia Huerta Victorino that shocked her family, friends and school counselor. Yes, she had struggled for years with learning disabilities and a series of losses. Yes, she was angry and got into fights at school. Yes, she had been identified as depressed and hospitalized in November 2003, when a teacher caught her scribbling a list of "top ten ways to kill yourself and love yourself." She received weekly counseling sessions for several months and a psychiatrist recommended medication. Her father, saying that both counseling and medications were against his beliefs and not realizing the seriousness of her depression, withdrew her from treatment. Her complaints—that she didn't have any friends and no one liked her at school—seemed fairly typical of teenage angst. When she hanged herself, leaving a note that said "Sorry for what I did, but I had to. No one liked me anymore . . . P.S. I was 15", all of those who knew and loved her struggled to understand why. What emerged was a pattern of loss and depression that had been expressed as anger, irritability and aggression, too often masking the sadness and hopelessness that had consumed the young girl.

Sometimes loss and depression can be temporarily obscured by seemingly positive events. Mark and Cheryl Miller, profiled in a recent *New York Times Magazine* article on teenagers and antidepressants, thought a move from a small town to a nearby upscale neighborhood in Kansas City would provide even more advantages for their children. Both Jenny, fifteen, and Matt, thirteen, were excited about the move. But while Jenny thrived at her new high school, Matt struggled at his new middle school. He had difficulty making friends. His mother later observed that "the kids just weren't letting him in." His grades fell. At first, his parents thought it was just a sign of normal adjustment problems to middle school. When his classroom behavior became problematic, however, they sought treatment with a child psychiatrist who prescribed the antidepressant Zoloft. Mark became restless and agitated and had some angry outbursts. Less than a week after he began taking the medication, Mark hanged himself. His stunned and grieving parents then began a long and heartbreaking inquiry, not only into the events leading up to his death in 1997, but also into the role that Zoloft may have played in their son's suicide.

These three teens highlight, in two cases, tragically, the serious nature of teenage depression, the importance of early diagnosis and treatment, and the difficulty in making this diagnosis, as well as increasing concern about how antidepressant medications may be contributing to some teenage suicides.

Recent statistics show that although one in five young people have mental health problems and one in ten have serious emotional problems, relatively few of these—about 30 percent—receive treatment. The consequences of undiagnosed or untreated adolescent depression can be grim.

• Many experts in adolescent development and behavior see depression as a contributing factor to a host of adolescent problems, including eating disorders, drug and alcohol abuse, truancy and other difficulties at school, sexual risk taking, pregnancy, running away from home and suicide.

• Suicide is the third leading cause of death—after accidents and homicides—for fifteen to twenty-four year olds. It is the sixth leading cause of death for young people five to fourteen.

• A recent study by the National Institute of Mental Health revealed that 4.9 percent of nine to seventeen year olds surveyed showed signs of major depression and that this depression often co-occurred with anxiety disorders or physical illnesses, such as diabetes.

• Other studies have found that up to 14 percent of young people will experience an episode of major depression by their fifteenth birthday, with girls significantly more at risk for depression after the age of sixteen.

• A 2002 Brown University study found that parents often don't recognize symptoms of depression in their adolescents, even when the parents have good communication with their children.

• Gay and lesbian youth have a two-to-threefold risk of suicide and are at far greater risk for depression.

• Gender differences in depression are becoming disturbingly apparent, with girls having much more difficulty with depression in adolescence, according to a growing number of studies. This difficult passage into adolescence and early adulthood can leave lasting scars on the lives and the psyches of an entire generation of young women.

The studies and statistics are startling, but the individual stories behind these can be even more unsettling. The young people who figure into these statistics come from all communities, all socioeconomic levels, a variety of home situations, anybody's family. What they tend to have in common is depression. Feeling helpless and hopeless, many teenagers are using alcohol or drugs as self-medication. Pregnancy and/or sexual acting out, which can be not only life-changing, but also life-threatening in this age of AIDS, can seem like an antidote to the loneliness and isolation many teenagers feel. Truancy, running away, eating disorders and attempted suicide are often desperate cries for help.

When a teenager in your own family is experiencing such a crisis, the statistics become relatively meaningless. Trapped in a cycle of anger, confusion, fear and despair, parents and teens may all feel increasingly helpless and terribly alone.

I have seen this many times over, both in my work as a journalist and, later on, as a psychotherapist. Early in my career, I was an editor for *TEEN* magazine and an advice columnist for *Seventeen.* I had occasion to meet many troubled teenagers and their families—some struggling together, some very much alone.

There was fourteen-year-old Wendy, whom I interviewed at a shelter for teenage runaways in St. Louis. Wendy's parents had divorced and remarried—and it appeared that neither set of remarried parents really wanted her. So she had run away, and after only a short time living on the streets, had been the victim of an attempted strangulation. Purple bruises were evident on her neck as she drew her blanket around her like a cocoon and tried to explain why she had run away from home four times in the past two months. "I'm no good to anyone," she said quietly, staring at the floor. "I get upset and fuss at home and it causes trouble for everyone. I had to run away to save my parents' marriages."

One of the first patients I saw as a psychotherapy intern, Bryan, also fourteen, was caught between a severely depressed father dying of diabetic complications who had made frequent suicide attempts and a mother who distanced herself from the ongoing crisis at home with her work and her daily aerobics classes. Bryan struggled to care for his father while trying to cope with the pressures of adolescence. He was angry about being in treatment "because my parents are the crazy ones, not me!" And he was depressed: depressed over the seeming indifference of his mother, depressed over his inability to rescue his father. He wondered who he was, what he could become and whether any of his dreams for himself and his future were truly possible. We worked together, off and on, for four years—through his depression, his anguish over his father's death when he was seventeen, his ambivalence toward his mother and his growing hope for an independent future.

And there was Tai, who perhaps more than any other troubled teen, touched my life and my understanding of teenage depression. Bright, talented and personable, Tai was an "A" student, a promising ballet dancer and a model child. Even as she approached adolescence, her episodes of moodiness and rebellion were mild and only occasional. But everything changed for Tai during the second semester of her freshman year of high school. Her mother broke her hip in an auto accident, and many new household responsibilities fell on Tai as she took on a major role in helping her mother through a long convalescent period. During this difficult time, her beloved thirteen-year-old cat died and her best friend moved away. Initially, Tai seemed to cope well. She wrote to her friend, was gentle and caring with her mother and never said much about the cat. But there were changes—gradual at first and then accelerating into a crisis. She started spending most of her free time alone in her room and lost interest in her friends. She became increasingly sullen and snappish. Within six months, she was refusing to go to school, sleeping all day and staying up all night, pacing and crying. She lost twenty pounds, quit ballet and starting talking about suicide.

Unfortunately, Tai's story is not at all unusual. What made Tai unique for me was the fact that she is my younger sister. I am ten years older than she is, and during her crisis as a teen I began to see teenage depression from a new perspective: not as an objective professional, but as a concerned, sometimes despairing, family member. I watched, alarmed, and tried to help as Tai slipped further into deep depression and as our parents became more frightened and bewildered. Their initial impulse to punish her behavior vanished and, for months, they were completely at a loss to understand and to cope with this much-loved child who had suddenly become a stranger.

Finally, with the help of a skilled and sensitive therapist, Tai recovered from her episode of depression. But her crisis was costly in many ways. She never went back to high school, although she did pass an equivalency exam. Her dreams for a career in dance were derailed by the lost years and lost confidence.

From the perspective of time, however, some positive life events have emerged from that long-ago crisis. Well into young adulthood, Tai's memories of caring for her mother inspired her to return to school and to seek a career as a registered nurse. She brings unique compassion into this work she loves. Tai also has insights into teenage depression that many parents don't have—and has used her unique perspective to guide her own daughter Nicky, now fifteen, lovingly along her adolescent passage. Nicky is the healthy beneficiary of the lessons that her mother learned during a painful adolescence.

Still, it hurts to look back. Tai wishes that she had been more in touch with her feelings when she was a teen and that she had been able to ask for help early on. She wishes that our parents, now long deceased, had recognized the early warning signs of trouble and sought appropriate help before her depression escalated to a life-changing crisis. She wishes that she hadn't had to endure so much pain for so long.

Our parents' initial denial, confusion and helplessness, however, are common and understandable parental reactions to teenage depression. It's sometimes hard to spot clinical depression in the midst of "normal" adolescent angst. In many instances, a depressed teenager will seem irritable, moody and rebellious—as teenagers can often be. How can a parent tell what is a temporary stage and what is a crisis? Why do so many teenagers suffer from depression? Can it be prevented? How can the parents of a depressed teen deal with their own feelings of shock, fear, anger and guilt? And how can a parent help a deeply depressed adolescent? When is it time to seek outside help—and what kind of help is most beneficial?

This book—with insights and guidelines from a variety of mental health experts, parents and teens themselves—is designed to help concerned parents who may be asking such questions.

Parents are of vital importance to a depressed teenager. As a parent, you can be your child's best initial source of help if you understand the dynamics, the causes, the symptoms and the most constructive ways of dealing with your teenager's depressive crisis. By taking early and appropriate action, you can help your son or daughter to avoid or overcome serious depression and thus prevent him or her from becoming yet another tragic statistic.

Part I

FACING FACTS ABOUT
TEENAGE DEPRESSION

CHAPTER

1

Teenage Depression: What Is It?

"Why live? Why die? To keep on living an empty life takes patience from an empty person. . . ."

These words were taken from the diary of Vivienne Loomis, a bright, attractive, well-loved fourteen-year-old whose suicide in 1973 shocked and bewildered both family and friends. And yet Vivienne *had* given warning signals for months. She had confided her feelings to close friends. She had written letters to her teachers.

Yet her signals were not taken seriously. She was so bright. She had so much to live for. She *couldn't* be serious about taking her own life. But, tragically, Vivienne was serious. Although she died more than thirty years ago, Vivienne Loomis is a timeless example of the tragedy of teen suicide.

Although some depressed, even suicidal, teenagers come from extremely troubled backgrounds with a lifetime of difficulties at home and at school, the vast majority of depressed teens are not without resources, support or love. They simply find, for a variety of reasons, that they're feeling overwhelmed by a sensation of hopelessness and helplessness. It can happen to the best and the brightest of young people.

Ron Wells, for example, was a seventeen-year-old with many accomplishments already behind him and a bright future ahead. Academically gifted, popular, handsome and athletic, he had recently graduated at the top of his high school class and had been accepted to a highly competitive Ivy League college.

That summer, poised between high school and college, Ron began to change. He became reclusive, moody and apathetic. He ate very little and talked even less, snappishly dismissing his puzzled parents' concern and refusing to take calls from friends. When he did talk, it was to complain about life being a burden, about feeling empty, down, depressed.

His parents were bewildered. "But you have everything, and now you're going to the college you've always dreamed of attending!" his father replied with more than a hint of impatience. "What does it take? What more could you want?"

The question went unanswered until a family friend suggested that Ron and his parents seek therapy together. Gradually the pieces of the puzzle began to fit: Ron was feeling a loss of lifelong goals in the wake of achieving them, and his long-term goals—to go to medical school and to build a private practice in sports medicine—seemed so far away; he was feeling scared about holding his own in the competitive college environment and wondered if his days of being a star student and outstanding student leader were behind him; he was sad about leaving his parents and friends in Oregon for college in the East; he experienced the weight of parental expectations to be the best and brightest, and sometimes suspected, as they celebrated his latest achievement, that he was loved for what he did, not for the person he was. Ron was also nervous about what would happen when he left home. His parents had been having some marital difficulties, and deep down he felt somewhat responsible for keeping them together. Would the family fall apart if he left Oregon to follow his educational dreams a continent away? And Ron had a family history of depression: His maternal grandfather had suffered from recurring bouts of depression all of his life, and his mother, Pam, had experienced similar difficulties during Ron's childhood and adolescence.

As therapy helped to reveal Ron's concerns and difficulties as he faced the transition from high school to college, and as his family history of depression emerged, his depression became more understandable—and treatable. With a lot of work, commitment and love, Ron and his parents began to communicate and work through most of the issues behind his depressed mood. He subsequently left for college and experienced continued success. His parents resolved many of their difficulties in marriage counseling, and at last report the family was doing well.

If you have a depressed teenager—or know one—Ron's story may have some familiar elements: the irritability, the snappishness, the withdrawal, the confused parents who wonder why a young person with all the advantages of youth, vitality and a lifetime of opportunities ahead would feel so hopeless. Sure, adolescence is not a breeze. Friends can be fickle. Growing and changing bodies can be awkward. There is that constant, baffling mixture of yearning for security and pushing toward independence that makes a child want to be nurtured one day and proclaim his autonomy the next. But to an adult these conflicts seem temporary and minor, and they pale in comparison to the advantages of youth. Depression and youth seem utterly incongruous.

But depression does happen in the young—even infants and children. Until the last two decades, the mental-health professions, dominated by traditional psychoanalytic theories, held to the belief that serious, ongoing depression could not exist before the formation of the idealized self-image (also called the superego), a developmental stage usually not reached until well into adolescence. A youngster's personality was not deemed sufficiently mature to suffer serious depression. This belief resulted in a delay of research into the phenomenon of childhood and adolescent depression. But times are changing. There has been a dramatic increase in research into and knowledge about adolescent depression in the past decade. As a result, more and more professionals are recognizing the fact that young people can become depressed.

What are we talking about when we discuss "teenage depression"?

That's an important question and one we'll be discussing over the next few chapters as we look at the symptoms of depression in adolescents, how depressed teenagers differ from depressed adults and how, although the signs and symptoms of teenage depression can appear quite similar to "normal" teenage rebellion, a concerned parent can distinguish predictable teenage turbulence from serious depression.

Depression is often used as a sort of catchall phrase to describe a variety of symptoms. Sigmund Freud saw depression as a reaction to early losses and separations, a result of rage and guilt turned inward. Today we might describe depression as the result of a complex mix of social, psychological and/or physical factors that can act on a person's nervous system, triggering sadness, hopelessness and self-deprecating thinking and behavior. For some people depression comes in the wake of a major loss or setback. For others the reasons are not so clear-cut. For some, depression can be a lifelong illness that comes and goes in a recurring cycle.

Distressed adolescents may suffer from a variety of different types of depression, varying considerably in severity, duration and impact on the teenager's life.

Types of Teenage Depression

DEPRESSED MOOD

These feelings of sadness and unhappiness may occur as the result of a specific event in a teenager's life. Maybe it's a setback such as not making a sports team or cheerleading squad or winning an academic honor. Maybe it's a response to loss—the loss of a boyfriend or girlfriend. It may be triggered by parental divorce, a friend moving away, the death of a pet or some other loss that is significant to the teenager.

Grief for the loss of a loved one is quite different. Grief is mourning the loss of a significant relationship. When a grieving person also experiences feelings of worthlessness, withdrawal from friends and family, a variety of physical symptoms or feelings of sadness that prevent that person from functioning, grief is being complicated by depression.

A depressed mood may occur suddenly in response to a loss situation and may either be brief or persist for an extended period of time. Depressed mood is usually quite identifiable as sadness and unhappiness.

MAJOR DEPRESSION

The teen suffering from major depression must have suffered from five or more specific symptoms for at least two weeks (and in a way that interferes with his or her previous functioning). These symptoms include:

1. Depression or irritability most of the day, nearly every day.
2. Loss of or diminished interest in activities he or she may have enjoyed previously.

3. Significant weight loss or gain, diminished or increased appetite. In teens, the failure to make expected weight gains as the body grows can be an important sign of trouble.
4. Feelings of restlessness or being slowed down.
5. Daily fatigue or loss of energy.
6. Sleep disturbances—either sleeping too much or too little.
7. Feelings of worthlessness or excessive or inappropriate guilt on a daily basis.
8. Diminished ability to concentrate or make decisions nearly every day.
9. Suicidal thoughts, plans and/or attempts.

Largely depending on how much the teenager's life is impaired by depressive symptoms, a major depression can be classified as "mild," "moderate" or "severe."

DYSTHYMIA

Dysthymia is a form of chronic depression that is diagnosed only when a child or teenager has experienced depressed or irritable moods consistently over a period of one year without more than two months without symptoms. Associated symptoms include decreased or increased appetite, sleeping too much or not enough, low energy, low self-esteem, poor concentration, impaired decision-making ability and feelings of hopelessness.

It is quite common for other problems to occur concurrently with dysthymia. About one-third to two-thirds of teens with dysthymic disorder have an anxiety disorder as well. Twenty to thirty percent of dysthymic teens have attention deficit disorder (ADD). Others may show signs of eating disorders, substance abuse or behavioral problems.

DOUBLE DEPRESSION

If a major depression and dysthymia coincide, this is called double depression. The teen with double depression can exhibit more severe depressive symptoms over a longer period of time and is at greater risk for suicide.

BIPOLAR DISORDER

Classified, like depression, as a mood disorder, bipolar disorder can also be a somewhat different manifestation of teenage depression.

Here moods alternate between manic, or abnormally elevated, moods— marked by agitation, decreased need for sleep, inflated self-esteem, incessant talking, increased activity level and excessive involvement in pleasurable but sometimes risky activities—and major depression.

There is a more chronic form of bipolar disorder called *cyclothymia.* The adolescent diagnosed with this disorder must have had at least a year of not being without either manic or major depression symptoms for more than two months.

As you read the symptoms and descriptions, perhaps with growing alarm, you may find yourself wondering, "Why does this happen?"

You're not alone. The more we learn about teenage depression, the more adults—parents, educators, physicians, mental-health professionals and others who care for and about young people—wonder why. Why does depression strike some young people just when their lives are so full of promise and potential?

2

Why Does Adolescent Depression Happen?

"Why? Why are teenagers more depressed today? We all know that it's tough being a teenager, but we made it without all this trouble. What's behind all this depression?"

This question has been asked by parents, by television and radio hosts, by educators and others concerned with teenagers in the decade since the first edition of this book, *Coping with Teenage Depression,* was published in 1982. It is a question with several answers.

When today's parents were growing up in the fifties and sixties, there were undoubtedly depressed teenagers who, like many of today's teens, attempted to anesthetize their sorrows in alcohol or overeating or sexual acting out. Those teens had a particular kind of pain, since their depression went largely undiagnosed. This was a time when experts believed that young adolescents were not emotionally developed enough to experience true depression. It was a time when getting psychotherapy carried a certain stigma and relatively few depressed adolescents got professional help. It was a time when a depressed teenager might be told, "Cheer up! These are the best years of your life! Wait until you're an adult and have real problems!"

So many of yesterday's depressed teenagers struggled along as best they could. Some overcame or learned to live with their depression with time and self-care. Some, like Vivienne Loomis (whose diary entry began the last chapter), did not survive.

Teenagers have always been vulnerable to depression for a variety of reasons. Loss, change and parental depression are among the major factors to be covered at length in this chapter. But today's teens face an additional challenge: They're growing up in a world quite different from that of their parents' youth.

The parents of today's teens came of age in an era of economic growth and optimism. Even if our parents struggled to make ends meet (usually on one salary), even if their marriages bore no resemblance to the Cleavers', we grew up with the hope and expectation that we would do better than our parents. Even if we worried about the Bomb, we lived in a nation that had won its wars, including the war in space to put the first man on the moon. Even as we protested Vietnam, we had hope for changing the system. And our sexual awakenings came at a time of unprecedented freedom.

Today's teens are coming of age at a time of declining national power, of corporate downsizing, when more and more families are beset by unemployment and careers are derailed by circumstance. It is a time when college costs are soaring and a college degree is no longer a guaranteed ticket to the good life. Some 40 percent of today's teens will grow up in homes divided by parental divorce. There has been a steady erosion of family earnings. A study by the Center for the Study of Social Policy found that between 1979 and 1990, the real median income of families with children fell by 5 percent. To keep families afloat economically, more mothers are working outside the home: 61 percent in 1990 versus 53 percent in 1980. Families have less time, less money and more stress today—and fewer backup resources for nurturing their children.

These young people face stress in the schools, as well—with resources dwindling and campus violence and harassment increasing—and their sexual awakening comes in the age of AIDS, when sex can kill.

Today's internet savvy teens have a front-row seat to a shrinking and dangerous world community. In our post-9/11 era, with instant images of terrorism on the Internet and nightly television news, teens are growing up in a world made more fearful. Middle East conflicts rage on and today's teens express a very real fear of being drawn into the battles. They see, more than other generations, the fragility of life, not only in the face of international terrorism, but also as they are confronted with instant, vivid images of natural disasters—like the horrific tsunami that swept through Asia in late December 2004.

In summary, teens today feel less safe, less empowered and less hopeful than we did a generation ago.

Superimposed on this scenario are the factors that have historically made teenagers vulnerable to depression. Usually, teenage depression is not due to one factor alone but to a combination of stressors.

"Factors such as a parental divorce or family relocation can be significant losses to a teenager, but they are not usually enough *in isolation* to bring about severe depression in a teen," contends Dr. Calvin Frederick, chief of Emergency Mental Health at the National Institute of Mental Health and professor of psychiatry at George Washington University.

The following stressors are the most commonly cited in connection with teenage depression. If your child is experiencing several of these in combination, he or she could be at risk for serious depression.

Family Stresses

PARENTAL DEPRESSION

If a teenager has a depressed parent, this is a major risk factor for adolescent depression.

What puts the teenager at risk? "It is a multitude of factors," says Dr. Anne C. Petersen of the Institute for Child Development and the department of pediatrics at the University of Minnesota. "This includes genetic, predisposition to depression, the emotional unavailability of parents because of depression, dysfunctional parent-child interactions and marital conflicts."

"A depressed parent may not be able to see beyond their own needs," says Dr. Gabrielle Carlson, a nationally known expert on childhood and adolescent depression. "They may have a chronic 'Who cares?' or 'Oh, shut up!' attitude toward their children. From a commonsense point of view, this has to have an impact on the child, especially if he or she has no other resources to turn to."

The genetic factor in depression is one that has fascinated researchers for years. There is increasing evidence that some depression can have a biochemical basis. Research into brain functioning has revealed that vital information regulating feelings, thoughts and behavior is transmitted to brain cells by the nervous system through the release of chemical substances called neurotransmitters. Released at nerve terminals, these chemicals cause an electrical chain reaction of sorts from one nerve ending to another. In the part of the brain that is associated with emotions, the brain-function neurotransmitters are amino acid compounds called biogenic amines; they include serotonin and norepinephrine. Some scientists believe that an imbalance of these chemicals in the brain might be linked to depression in some people. Studies have found that an imbalance of serotonin may lead to depressive symptoms such as irritability, anxiety and sleep problems. Fatigue and depressed mood can result from an imbalance of norepinephrine. A number of antidepressant medications work by altering the action of amines in the brain, thus correcting existing chemical imbalances. Some believe that a tendency to have an imbalance of the brain's neurotransmitters may be an inherited characteristic.

A number of studies have provided some evidence to support the theory that depression—or a tendency toward depression—can have, in part, a genetic basis.

For example, at the 1993 North American Conference on Adoptable Children, Dr. Anu Sharma of the Search Institute in Minnesota reported early findings of a 775-family study that revealed that teens adopted as infants were more likely to feel sad or anxious and that the birth mother's depression rating predicts the adopted teen's depression score (and her alcohol use, drug use and sexual behavior strongly predict similar behaviors in her child). On the other hand, an adoptive mother's behavior and depression rating have "virtually zero" correlation with her adopted teen's behaviors.

Other studies of adopted children have found that even if raised in adoptive homes where the parents are not depressed, the adoptees have a threefold risk for depression if their biological relatives suffered from depression.

Studies of twins raised apart also have provided interesting comparisons of genetic versus environmental influences. It has been found that if one identical twin suffers from a depression disorder, the other twin has a 60 to 70 percent chance of sharing the disorder—even if the two were raised separately.

Dr. Donald McKnew and Dr. Leon Cytryn, authors of *Why Isn't Johnny Crying?,* have been studying the children of manic-depressive parents for some years, following the offspring from childhood through young adulthood. They found that the incidence of depression in the children of parents *without* manic depression was about 10 percent, while 30 to 50 percent of the children whose parents suffered from manic depression were found to be depressed.

In his studies of the genetic roots of depression, Dr. George Winokur of the University of Iowa has found that a group of patients with a family history of depression consistently scored highest on hormone tests revealing endocrine abnormality.

While there is much research yet to be done to clarify genetic influences on depression, much current study points to the possibility that a predisposition to depression can be inherited and, when activated by a mix of environmental and psychosocial factors, can result in a teen's depression.

FAMILY CRISIS

There are certain family crises that can become major factors in teenage depression. Parental divorce is certainly one of these. In Dr. Judith Wallerstein's ongoing California Children of Divorce study, she found that five years after their parents had split up, more than one-third of the children were experiencing moderate or severe depression. Ten years after the divorce, a significant number still appeared to be troubled underachievers.

Other studies present troubling statistics about children of divorce: Girls are at greater risk for early sexual activity and pregnancy as well as for dropping out of high school. Boys are at still greater risk for dropping out of high school than girls and are more likely to engage in aggressive behavior. And a 1992 study on depression and self-esteem of teens whose parents were divorced found that children of divorced parents have higher levels of depression and lower self-esteem—as well as lower grade-point averages in school—than their peers whose parents are not divorced.

Remarriage of one or both parents, while a new beginning for the parent, can become an emotional crisis for the teenager. The National Commission on Children recently reported that children and teenagers living in stepfamilies were more likely to say that they felt lonely or depressed. Why? The commission found that remarried parents, perhaps investing more energy in efforts to build a new marriage and make it work, invest less time in their children than do parents in intact families or single parents.

A study by Dr. Lawrence Kurdek of Wright State University found that girls who were living in families with a stepfather were at highest risk for academic difficulties, low self-esteem, health problems, drug use and other symptoms of depression, while the boys most at risk were those living with mothers who had been divorced multiple times.

Unemployment and/or financial stresses can also have a major impact on teenagers. Teens can feel considerable pressure and stress when a parent is unemployed. The stress is particularly high in children of white-collar workers who have not previously experienced layoffs and who have always been financially comfortable, even affluent.

"It's pretty bad," says Jennifer, fifteen, whose father, an aerospace engineer, was laid off eight months ago and whose mother, a librarian, fears losing her job in the wake of state spending cuts for libraries. "My parents are really tense. They yell at each other a lot and at me even more. We never do anything fun. I had to give up my ballet and voice lessons. I've tried to earn money by babysitting, but with a lot of people out of work around here, people are mostly staying home. It's so depressing. What is the most depressing is that here my parents did all the things they keep telling me I should do—like they did well in school, went to college, worked hard . . . and now look. We might even lose our house if Dad doesn't get a job soon. Whenever the phone rings, we get scared it's some person demanding money. Sometimes I just cry, thinking about how good life used to be."

Marta, now nineteen and a community-college student, says that she will never forget when her father lost his aerospace job. "He was in a total panic," she says, her eyes filling with tears at the memory. "He would get out the want ads, and because he got so depressed reading them, he'd hand them to me and say, 'Look and see if there are any engineering jobs in there. Find me a job, honey!' It made me feel so scared! He never did get another job. My mother, who is a nurse, went back to work and has supported the family since then, and now he's pretty much out of it—drinking too much and watching TV all day. It has changed me a lot. I feel down and scared a lot of the time, like nothing in life will ever be for sure. I used to dream about being an actress or a writer, but now I'm studying to be a nurse, like my mom, because I always want to be able to get a job. I see dreams as a luxury I can't afford."

A family illness—of a parent, a sibling or a grandparent—can also have an impact on a teenager, who may have myriad feelings, including fear, anxiety, grief and guilt mixed in with his or her depression over the family situation.

In summary, while adolescents may seem at times quite removed from family issues, as part of the family system they are vulnerable to stresses, especially to trickle-down depression and anxiety.

FAMILY DYSFUNCTION

"Dysfunction" is an often-used word these days and simply means that something isn't working. In a family, it may be that family members aren't communicating well with one another. It may mean that one or more people in a family are abusing other family members physically, emotionally or sexually. It may mean that the family's style of behavior is not optimal for a teenager's needs as a growing young adult.

For example, in researching the role of family interactions on the onset of teenage depression, Dr. Steven Katz of Northwestern University Memorial Hospital notes that "parents of depressed adolescents are more hostile and critical and more controlling toward their adolescents as well as less responsible in general toward their depressed adolescents than are parents of normal adolescents. Depressive behavior and thinking develop in response to these chronic interpersonal patterns rather than in response to any isolated traumas."

French researcher Dr. Marie Choquet has found that teens can become depressed if their parents are overprotective and "suffocating," but teens are *most* depressed when their parents show a lack of interest in them.

Other studies in this country have concurred that some of the most depressed teens are those whose families prematurely launch them into independence before they have the emotional or practical skills to handle such freedom. Such teens tend to feel rejected and unloved instead of empowered.

HIGH PARENTAL EXPECTATIONS

Parental expectations, if they are communicated with love and if they are based in reality, can help to encourage a teen to be his or her best.

Some parents, however, voice expectations that feel, to the teen, impossible to meet, and some teens feel that parental love is conditional on achievement.

"I've been depressed and down on myself because I can't be what my parents want me to be," says Rick, sixteen, a high school junior with a slight learning disability. "My older brother was this super athlete and top student and they think he's perfect. My grades . . . I mean, I think that I work much harder in school than he did, but I don't get any credit for that. They just punish me for getting Cs and they think if I get a B that's no big deal, except it is for me. They expect me to be like my brother and I can't be—and they don't think I'm any good if I can't measure up. I feel like nothing I ever do will please them or make them proud. I wonder if they really love me. And I feel pretty much alone."

For Melissa, seventeen, a science-fair winner who is aiming for medical school, her parents' high expectations get in the way of praise she feels she needs. "They just expect me to be the best . . . always . . . and when I do win prizes or come out on top, it's no big deal to them," she says. "They just say, 'Of course you won. You're our daughter . . . our future doctor-in-the-family.' I know they mean well, but I'd like to hear them praise . . . oh, I don't know . . . my efforts or my self-discipline or my imagination—you know, the things that go into my successes—instead of just accepting my successes as their due. Sometimes I feel like messing up or running away just to shake them up. I wouldn't do that . . . but sometimes it's tempting. I really get depressed when I feel like I'm their little 'success object.' I don't think they even know or care about the *person* I am."

Psychosocial Stresses

REJECTION OR HARASSMENT BY PEERS

Teens who feel rejected by their peers are more likely to be depressed than those who feel they fit in with classmates.

Psychologist Antonius Cillessen of Duke University and a team of Dutch researchers found that peer rejection can generate a lifelong tendency toward depression. In his study of 231 Dutch schoolboys, Cillessen considered the question "Are kids rejected by peers because of an emotional problem, or do they develop emotional problems as a result of rejection?" He found that there was often interplay between the two. Those singled out for rejection were usually shy or, at the other extreme, those who were aggressive. Dr. Cillessen found that the rejected kids most at risk for later depression were the shy ones.

In a study of 750 fourth-graders, Dr. David A. Cole of Notre Dame University found the correlations between symptoms of depression and social and/or academic failures to be "substantially higher" than that reported in earlier studies. He found that such failures tended to have a cumulative effect on depression, with children who perceive themselves as losers in academic and/or social areas showing many more depressive symptoms.

GROWING UP FEMALE

In general, young adolescent girls are at much higher risk than boys for depression. This pattern can begin as early as the latter years of elementary school, when, studies have found, teachers and peers rate girls as more academically competent than boys, yet the girls themselves underrate their competence and attribute any school difficulties to lack of ability (as opposed to boys, who chalk school failures up to lack of effort).

A recent study by the American Association of University Women also found that teachers tend to undermine girls' educational opportunities by giving them less attention than boys and steering them away from science and technical courses. The study, which was conducted by the Wellesley College Center for Research on Women, also found that females are often stereotyped or ignored in many courses and that standardized tests are often full of gender-based biases.

Girls learn their lessons well. The trend toward devaluation of self is exacerbated as puberty begins. Statistically, girls' academic performance, especially in traditionally "male" areas such as math and science, tends to drop in adolescence as many girls feel the traditional double bind: feeling low self-esteem if they don't perform well in school, yet feeling low self-esteem if they do perform well academically and fail to get positive affirmation from peers, who tend to overvalue physical attributes such as thinness and prettiness in girls rather than competence or personality, two of the major popularity factors in adolescent boys. (This is mirrored in some magazines aimed at young girls. For example, a recent issue of *YM* featured an opinion poll "Do Guys Like Smart Girls?" and the vote was a unanimous "No!" A sample comment from a guy: "I don't find smart girls attractive.")

Girls are more likely to be adversely affected by sexual harassment at school, usually between the sixth and ninth grades. In a 1993 study released by the American Association of University Women Educational Foundation, 1,632 students in grades eight through eleven were surveyed. "There is an attitude of 'Boys will be boys,'" said Sharon Schuster, president of AAUW, when the report was released. "We haven't been aware how harmful it is, haven't recognized that girls are really impacted and that it makes a difference in how they do in school."

The survey found that 33 percent of girls who had been sexually harassed reported not wanting to attend school (versus 12 percent of all boys). More girls than boys reported feeling afraid and less confident about themselves because of sexual harassment.

Girls are also more likely to encounter other stresses in early adolescence. Statistically, parents of young adolescent girls are three times more likely to divorce than those of young adolescent boys. And the beginning of puberty in girls, which starts one to two years earlier than in boys, is more likely to coincide with the stressful switch to junior high, while boys usually go through puberty *after* making the adjustment from elementary school to junior high.

Girls who are early developers are at special risk for depression and low self-esteem. Dr. Anne Petersen of the University of Minnesota, who has conducted extensive research in this area, notes that "early developing girls steadily decline in body image even up to age seventeen, while early developing boys have very good body image. We have also found in our research that high stress such as sexual abuse or family conflicts can bring on puberty early in a girl, and this early development is its own risk factor for depression, poor body image and lower educational or occupational achievement. In general, girls are more depressed in early adolescence because they experience more challenging events during this time."

ISSUES WITH ETHNICITY

A recent study at UCLA revealed that while girls reported more depressive symptoms than males across all ethnicities, the differences between depressed adolescent males and females were less among Latinos. Researchers feel that physical changes of puberty, in particular, were triggers for stress and depression among Latino teens—especially in those whose development was either earlier or later than the physical changes of their peers. They concluded that, for Latino teens, nonconformity with peers might be more distressing to them than it is for white or African-American teens.

The UCLA researchers also found that Latino teens reported a greater variety of depressive symptoms. They concluded that, while it is possible that Latino adolescents were simply more likely to feel comfortable with revealing and discussing their depression than other teens, it seemed more likely that other factors—such as economic and other significant social stressors, such as racism and obstacles to education and lack of hope for the future were major contributing factors to the teens' depression. It was found, for example, that as family income decreased, the average level of teenage depression increased.

SEXUAL ORIENTATION

Gay and lesbian teenagers, or teens who think or fear that they may be homosexual, face special stresses in adolescence: the pain of feeling different from peers, of fearing rejection from parents and other family members as well as classmates, of enduring ridicule and harassment from classmates.

In the AAUW study on sexual harassment in the schools, 86 percent of the students said they would be "very upset" if called gay or lesbian. This was, in fact, the most upsetting form of sexual harassment for boys.

Recent government studies have found that teens struggling with their sexual orientation (and with the attendant harassment or rejection by peers, family conflict and feelings of isolation and hopelessness) are three times more likely than other teenagers to commit suicide. In a *New York Times* editorial, writer Sasha Alyson asked recently: "How many would still be alive if we had shown them that gayness and happiness were fully compatible?"

LEARNING DISABILITIES

Teens with learning disabilities such as dyslexia and attention deficit disorder (ADD) are also at high risk for depression. According to psychologist Benjamin Garber, learning disabilities are seriously underexamined as a cause of adolescent distress—with sometimes tragic consequences. "We now know that a learning disability is not just a school problem, but a life problem," he says.

"Children and teenagers with learning disabilities can get depressed because they can't do what their classmates can do," says Dr. Clarice J. Kestenbaum, director of training for the department of psychiatry at Columbia University's College of Physicians and Surgeons. "Self-esteem is intertwined with sense of self. If the adolescent is not successful in academic and/or social arenas, the traumas remain through adolescence and adulthood like old acne scars. And parental rejection of an 'imperfect' child may cause serious [emotional] injury. All children need parental admiration and approval."

Significant Losses

Loss can be due to death, divorce, separation or loss of an important friend or romantic interest. Loss can also be more subtle—the loss of childhood, of a familiar way of being, of goals through achievement or of boundaries and guidelines. These are some of the most common "loss traumas" that can be a factor in triggering depression in teenagers.

THE DEATH OF A LOVED ONE

The death of a parent or close family member is a major trauma for an adolescent. He or she may feel temporarily devastated by grief, guilt, panic and anger. If the young person is not able to express these feelings in a supportive atmosphere, depression may set in.

When John's twelve-year-old brother, David, died of cancer, he never shed a tear or showed any other outward signs of grieving. But in the weeks following his brother's death, John, thirteen, began getting into fights at school, withdrew from his friends and became alternately distant and angry with his parents. Bewildered, his parents took him to see the hospital social worker who had counseled the family throughout David's illness. It took several sessions both alone and with the family to help John begin to voice his feelings. He had not been able to cry, even though he was devastated by the loss of his brother, "because I'm walking around with a big, hurting lump inside me. I tried to pound it out by fighting, but it didn't work."

Finally, with support from his parents and therapist, John was able to cry and to voice other feelings such as guilt over his jealousy of David, who had received the lion's share of parental attention during his long illness. He was also able to voice his anger and grief over his brother's death and his fear that his parents sometimes wished that he, not David, had died.

The death of a parent can be devastating at a time when the teen is fighting for independence but still needs the parent very much. Terri was a week away from her fourteenth birthday when her father died suddenly of a heart attack. She cried continually, refused to go to school and lost ten pounds in three weeks following his death. She also started picking fights with her mother and younger brother, alternating between bouts of despair and bursts of anger. Finally, her worried and exhausted mother took her to the family doctor.

When the doctor gently asked Terri what she was feeling and how losing her father was affecting her, she began to cry. "We didn't get to say good-bye because he died at work," she sobbed. "I can't stand it. I didn't get a chance to tell him I loved him. We always got along great until this year, when I started wanting to be on my own more and I mouthed off to him a lot. I had a fight with him the night before he died about something that was just dumb. I feel like a terrible person. Now he'll never know I loved him. It's like nothing matters anymore. And I'm mad at God, too. Why did my dad have to die when I loved and needed him so much?"

Grief over the death of a friend also can be especially painful at a time when friends are so important. A friend's death is also a reminder of our own mortality. Guilt can take its toll, too. If the friend died in an accident or by suicide, the teenager may be plagued by "If only's," asking over and over why he or she wasn't there when needed. These "if only's" are a way of denying helplessness in the face of death. Denial, rather than acceptance, is often a forerunner of depression.

The death of a pet is frequently a major crisis for a young adolescent—one that is too often minimized. Some youngsters become very close to their pets even as they begin to pull away from the family in their quest for independence.

When Tai's thirteen-year-old cat, whom she had received as a kitten for her first birthday present, died, she sank into a major depression. There were other stressors in Tai's life, but the loss of her cat pushed her over the edge into depressive illness. "I didn't feel I could talk to my parents and I didn't have any real friends . . . except my cat, Edie. I used to tell her my problems. She would put her paws around my neck, lick my tears away and purr. She always loved me no matter what. When I lost her, it felt like I had lost . . . everything."

Tai's feelings of loss and desperation were heightened by the fact that she was afraid and embarrassed to tell anyone how much the cat had meant to her. It seemed that her family took the death rather casually. After her only school friend had moved away and her mother had been seriously injured in an accident, requiring special care at home, the loss of Edie was the final, unbearable loss to Tai. She never said much to anyone, but her behavior began to change abruptly after she lost her pet. She became even more isolated, refusing to go to school and sleeping all day. She lost interest in ballet, stopped eating and started talking about suicide.

"It seemed, quite simply, like the end of the world to me," Tai remembers. "I didn't see any real reason to live. I'll never forget that, and as a parent now, I would never, never underestimate that loss if it were to happen to my own daughter."

SEPARATION FROM A LOVED ONE

Death, of course, is not the only loss that can cause depression. Separation from an important person can also be a factor in adolescent depression. This separation often comes about as the result of divorce, when a parent moves out of the house and, in some sense, out of the child's life. But such separations also occur as the result of constant business travel, long tours of duty in the service or a parental jail term. In some ways a separation can be even more painful than the death of a loved one.

"Separation from a vital love object is a major stress factor," says Dr. Donald McKnew, a child psychiatrist and one of the nation's best known and most respected researchers on the subject of childhood and adolescent depression. "We have found that the damage seems to be greater in a coming-and-going situation—when the loved one drops in and out of a child's life—than it is in the single, final separation that death brings."

The fact of death, after all, is nonnegotiable. It must be faced and life must go on without the lost loved one. But when an important person drops in and out of a youngster's life, the teen may suffer from an ongoing cycle of hope, disappointment, rejection and despair.

After her parents' divorce, for example, Tammy began running away to the homes of friends for a day or two at a time. Her grades dropped and she spent a lot of time alone in her room, sulking and crying. During a conference with Tammy's teacher, her mother observed that these episodes were often linked with her father's behavior. Despite liberal visitation rights, Tammy's father had almost dropped out of her life. He seldom called and almost never visited. It was usually Tammy who initiated the contact with her father. She felt terribly rejected by his long silences, coming to the conclusion that she was no longer loved or valued. But just when she was beginning to adjust to the fact that her father was gone, he would reappear with presents and promises of a closer, ongoing relationship and more frequent fun times together. Tammy's hopes would soar as he would make all kinds of plans for future get-togethers, only to be disappointed once again as her father totally disappeared from her life for months at a time. This cycle of hope, rejection and continual loss was, as subsequent counseling revealed, a major contributing factor to Tammy's depression.

Separation from friends and from one's roots due to a family move is a loss that can be a major stressor and help to push a teenager into depression.

Fourteen-year-old Melanie, for example, lost interest in hobbies and school and started sleeping a lot after her family moved from New Jersey to San Francisco. Her mother, worried that something might be physically wrong with Melanie, took her to see Dr. Charles Wibbelsman, an adolescent medicine specialist.

"There was nothing physically wrong with Melanie, but in talking with her I discovered that the family move had separated her from her best friend—a very significant person in her life—and she was greatly affected by this," says Dr. Wibbelsman. "Adults may tend to minimize such a loss. We know we can keep in touch, meet new friends and take care of ourselves. But these facts aren't obvious to the inexperienced teenager. A close friend is such a salient part of his or her life. Also, such partings are usually the result of a parental choice or transfer. When someone else makes the decision to move, the teenager suffers not only the loss of a friend, but also the sense of lacking control over his or her destiny. Some kids who do not have roots and whose parents move frequently have problems with peer relationships and are subject to periodic or chronic depression."

A romantic breakup, too, can be particularly devastating to a teenager, whose feelings are so new and intense and who does not yet know that one can survive the loss of a love, learn and grow from the experience and some-day love again.

LOSS OF A FAMILIAR WAY OF BEING

Adolescence brings a number of physical and psychosocial changes, all of which mean growth and loss.

"Depression is, to some extent, a part of normal adolescent development because in growing and developing, the young person experiences loss," says Dr. Richard C. Brown, director of Adolescent Health Services at San Francisco General Hospital. "This involves loss of childhood and family-centered life. In forming strong new ties with their friends and questioning family values and traditions, teens begin to separate from their families. They are making new commitments to new friends, feeling love and affection outside the family and seeing themselves as separate from the parents. Their bodies are changing, too, and these internal changes combined with social changes can make this a time of disequilibrium. The teenager is losing the comfort of dependence and the simplicity of being a child. As a result, the teenagers (and their parents, too) may be in a state of mourning."

Thirteen-year-old Kyra, for example, was distressed to find that even though she was growing to prefer the company of her friends most of the time, her parents were also becoming a bit more distant. She had always been especially close to her father, enjoying the outings, games and wrestling matches with him. As she began to develop physically, however, her father stopped the wrestling matches and, in fact, stopped touching her at all. He seemed a little uncomfortable around Kyra now that she was no longer physically a child.

Kyra saw this distance as rejection and as a huge loss. Her sadness and anger were evident when she told her school nurse, "I feel like either killing myself or tearing-up the photography book Dad gave me for Christmas—just to show him how I feel!"

LOSS OF SELF-ESTEEM

Depreciation, rejection and the inability to live up to high parental expectations can cause a significant loss of self-esteem and trigger depression in adolescents.

Teenagers, who are living through so many physical, social and emotional changes, are newly aware of their shortcomings and limitations and may be especially sensitive to criticism or rejection—obvious or implied, real or imagined. And teens' testing of boundaries, rules, ideas and behaviors may tax parental tolerance to the breaking point, making them easy targets for criticism.

"Teenagers are masters (often perceptive and accurate) at criticizing and expressing contempt," says Dr. Lee Robbins Gardner, a New Jersey psychiatrist. "However, they are simultaneously supersensitive to criticism, from parents especially. They need a lot of tact and small doses of criticism."

Also, certain patterns of rejection may escalate when a child reaches adolescence.

"Rejection often comes in the form of a blunt statement stressing the child's inadequacy," says Dr. McKnew. "Parents may be unaware of their own rejecting behavior. They may reject a fault or handicap in the child that they despise in themselves. A woman who doesn't feel good about her femininity may reject her daughter. A man may, for the same reasons, reject a son. Age can be a problem, too. Some parents are very good with infants, but reject their children as they get older and more independent. In this instance, the child can become very depressed and feel that he or she has let the parent down by growing up."

As Ken, a fourteen-year-old whose father died six months after Ken's birth, grew to prefer the company of his peers, his mother became angry and rejecting. He found himself torn between wanting to please his mother and wanting to please himself. His mother's labels, such as "selfish" and "ungrateful," increased his confusion and subsequent depression.

Dana was her father's favorite when she was little, cute and compliant. But when she began to develop her own interests and her own point of view, her father seemed to lose interest in her, favoring her younger brother instead. Dana is now struggling with feelings that she is a bad, unlovable person—even though no harsh or angry words have ever been spoken.

Jason, referred to a family therapist by his school counselor, has grown up with poor self-esteem. "Nothing I've ever done has ever been enough," he tells the counselor. "If I rake the leaves, Dad wants to know why I didn't clean the garage while I was at it. If I make an A-minus in school, my folks want to know why it wasn't an A and tell me I'm a failure. I'm getting interested in computers and am thinking about a college major in computer science or maybe engineering. But my parents have their hearts set on my being a doctor. Anything less makes me a second-class citizen or something. Nothing I accomplish is ever enough."

After speaking with Jason's parents, his counselor noted that their excessively high expectations for their son reflected their own feelings of inadequacy and their disappointment with their own career choices and financial status. Most parents, of course, want the best for their children. But Jason's parents felt that unless he was the best as *they* defined it, he was a failure.

Sometimes the patterns are less obvious. Dr. Gabrielle Carlson notes that in her practice at UCLA she encountered a teenage boy who was severely depressed and chronically suicidal, with very low self-esteem. "His father was a brain surgeon and his mother was a psychiatric social worker," she says. "I made the comment that I have never seen a chronically suicidal kid who didn't have family problems. They denied any problems. Yet as I watched the family talk with each other, I noticed that every time the boy said something, his mother would contradict him or discount what he was saying with a comment like, 'It *wasn't* that way. You misunderstood.' Nobody was listening to what the boy was saying."

The parent who doesn't listen is implying that what his or her child feels, thinks and says is not particularly important. Such a message can be a blow to a teen's often shaky self-esteem.

A crisis in self-esteem can also occur when a teenager is not allowed autonomy, is not trusted and is given little power over his or her own destiny. This saps self-esteem.

LOSS OF NORMALITY

Depression can be triggered by an illness or injury that sets a teenager apart from peers—temporarily or forever.

"Physical illness is a particular problem in adolescence because teenagers are so aware of and concerned with body image," says Dr. Gardner. "There is an extra emphasis on body image at this time and great emphasis, too, on all the changes the body is experiencing. Most teenagers are disturbed about at least one physical thing. It may be height, testicle size, breast development or even one pimple. There is a preoccupation with the body and any insult to it—even if it *seems* minor—may cause a major reaction."

Life is especially difficult for an adolescent with a chronic condition such as diabetes or epilepsy.

"We see quite a lot of depression in chronically ill adolescents," says Dr. Richard MacKenzie, director of the division of adolescent medicine at Children's Hospital of Los Angeles. "Teenagers with a chronic disease may feel inner turmoil about a disorder that separates them from their peers. There may be conflicts with parents about treatment routines and allowed activities. Parents may not trust the child's judgment. A chronic illness can also impede a teenager's emancipation from the family. All this sets the scene for serious depression. The teen's self-esteem is endangered tremendously."

For Christopher, seventeen, the epilepsy that developed after a head injury from a skateboarding accident when he was eleven was "the worst, the absolute worst, thing to ever happen to me."

Fighting tears, he looks away as he speaks, not wanting to show just how painful being different is for him. "There isn't an hour in any day that I don't think about epilepsy," he says. "I think about it when I see my friends all getting their driver's licenses and know that might not happen for me. I think about it when I'm at the beach with my friends and we're out in the water. Oh, I mustn't go out too far . . . might have a seizure. It has made it tough for me to have friends. Some have been great, but some think I'm weird because of the epilepsy, and they're like afraid to know me. I feel that epilepsy keeps me from being normal and being young."

Gayle's diabetes was diagnosed when she was ten, but the major conflicts about it and Gayle's serious depression over her illness didn't begin until she was in her early teens.

"I just got sick of having to be different," Gayle remembers. "I couldn't eat everything my friends ate. I had to follow—and still do—a strict meal schedule, which has always made my life less spontaneous than the lives of my friends. And my parents drove me bananas with their concern. They kept asking me, in front of my friends, even, "Have you eaten?" or "Have you tested your blood sugar?" And if we ate out, it was such a big deal. My mom would always make sure the chef knew that I was diabetic. God, I felt like they just should have made a sandwich-board sign with CAUTION: DIABETIC! on it for me to wear everywhere. I stopped trying to take responsibility for myself for a long time. I figured, 'If my parents are going to live life for me, I give up.' I felt for a long time like my parents sometimes used my diabetes to control me, to keep me from doing things I wanted to do. I was *so* depressed!"

A frightening health crisis and a sensitive yet strong-willed new doctor helped Gayle and her parents find a balance of power. From then on, Gayle has taken an increasing amount of responsibility for her own health and her life in general. Taking control of her medical condition has been a growing experience and a weapon against depression. "Now I feel like a normal person who just happens to have a medical problem that I can control," she says. "I don't feel strange, out-of-it and depressed that much anymore."

LOSS OF GOALS THROUGH ACHIEVEMENT

This sense of loss may be difficult to understand when it happens. The feeling strikes when things are going well, when a teenager has won a prize, made the team, met a challenge, finished a project, graduated or accomplished some other long-term goal. The fact behind this reaction to positive stress is that in achieving a goal one loses that goal. For a time the teen may wonder, "What now?" and feel a deep sense of loss.

"The senior year of high school can be a special problem for teenagers," Dr. Gardner observes. "There is a letdown. Bright kids who have fulfilled their dreams of admission to college are especially vulnerable. For years they've talked about and planned for college. Now they're in and feel frightened and conflicted when confronted with the fact that their dreams are becoming reality."

The reactions of others to the teen's achievement may heighten the youngster's sense of loss.

Two weeks after she won the "Best Actress" award in a statewide drama festival, Carole confided tearfully to a favorite teacher that winning the award meant more separateness than ever from her classmates. Some were obviously jealous and made cutting remarks; others seemed a bit in awe of her. This separateness—and the letdown involved in getting back to her regular routine after all the excitement of winning—added up to depression for Carole.

Jim, a math whiz, was elated when he was admitted to MIT. His excitement over college and his upcoming graduation gave way to confusion, disappointment and finally depression when he noticed the sudden coolness of Mr. Jackson, his math teacher and mentor for the past two years.

"This is not an unusual situation," says Dr. Gardner. "Teachers put a lot into the success of their students. Graduation can be a tremendous loss for a teacher, especially when kids express happiness at leaving and put down the school. There may be some role reversal as the kids overtake the teacher in certain ways. Physically, this may have happened earlier, but now the student may pass the teacher intellectually or in terms of achievement, and so teachers may be less than sympathetic."

All of these factors may combine to make some victories bittersweet and depression in the wake of triumph a real possibility.

LIMITED INNER RESOURCES FOR DEALING WITH FRUSTRATION AND LOSS

"Adolescents can be very fragile," observes Dr. Wibbelsman. "His or her life experience is so limited that the youngster has a great deal of difficulty finding workable solutions to a problem or crisis. Often teenagers don't have the experience and memories of coping constructively, or maybe even growing, through a difficult time."

The resulting sense of helplessness can lead to severe depression, even suicide. "When a teenager is suicidal, the three Hs—helplessness, haplessness and hopelessness—are usually present," says Dr. Calvin Frederick. "Events seem to be conspiring against the child, who feels helpless to deal with the problem. There seems to be no hope that things can be different. It is this loss of hope which can lead to serious depression and, possibly, suicide."

These feelings of helplessness and hopelessness can render adolescent depression potentially very dangerous. That is why it is so important for parents and other adults to understand the nature of teenage depression well enough to recognize or suspect it when it strikes a young son, daughter, relative or friend. It is imperative to realize that depression *does* happen to teenagers, even those who have everything going for them.

It is vital to admit that it could even happen to your child, that it might very well be part of the growing pains your son or daughter experiences during adolescence. And it may be comforting to know that recognition of these facts and the causes and sometimes unique symptoms of teenage depression is an important first step in helping your teenager find his or her way back from hopelessness.

Part II

IDENTIFYING TEENAGE DEPRESSION—THE SIGNS AND SYMPTOMS

3

Teenage Depression Is Different from Adult Depression

Teenage depression is elementally different in a number of ways from adult depression. These differences can be quite important. They make it difficult for parents or even health professionals to recognize depression in a teenager and to offer appropriate help and support.

What are some of the ways that teenage depression is different?

Teenagers Often Have Different Ways of Showing Depression

A depressed adult usually feels and looks sad and lethargic. A depressed teenager, on the other hand, may seem extremely angry, irritable and/or rebellious, with "acting out" behavior such as school problems, truancy, sexual risk taking, drinking, drug abuse, running away from home and psychosomatic symptoms quite common. These behavioral problems, which can mask depression, are not always indicative of underlying depression, but in many instances, they are.

"I believe that whenever you see an adolescent who has a constellation of symptoms and problems not fitting into a medical disorder or disease, depression should be considered as a cause," says Dr. Richard MacKenzie.

Dr. Richard Brown points out that it is the sometimes frenetic quality of teen depression that can be so misleading. "Hyperactivity, which can be a phobic reaction against depression, is often one of the characteristics of adolescent depression," he says. "The teen may *look* very nondepressed, but if you prick the surface of this hyperactivity, you will find in many instances that the young person is depressed."

Why do teenagers deal with their depression in these ways? Therapists who treat teenagers have a number of theories.

"Teenagers are being hit with so much so fast in the many hormonal, physical and social changes and tasks they face," says Shirley Lackey, a family therapist in La Mirada, California. "As a result, they may develop an intolerance of feeling and their emotions will only get discharged through actions."

A number of mental-health professionals believe that lack of verbal skills can be a major factor in a teen's acting-out behavior.

"One is not likely to see anything that looks like adult depression in an early or mid-adolescent—someone twelve to seventeen," contends Dr. Judith Davenport, a psychotherapist in private practice at the Center for Counseling and Psychotherapy in Santa Monica, California. "I feel this is so because cognitively, most kids' minds are not fully developed at this point. Many can't intellectually pinpoint and express what they're feeling. It's rare to hear a teenager come out and say, 'I feel depressed.' When this happens, it means 'I need help.' But generally teenagers have a great deal of ambivalence about their dependency needs versus their growing need for independence. For a teenager to admit that he or she needs help feels like regressing back to childhood."

And so depressed teens may cry for help indirectly through troublesome, even destructive, behavior and through physical symptoms.

Teenagers Elicit Different Responses to Their Depression

At least initially, an adult's sadness may bring sympathy from family and friends. A teenager's acting-out behavior tends to provoke alarm, anger, fear and frustration in those close to him or her.

"When Val was going through her crisis, depression was the last thing we thought of," admits her mother, Barbara. "She defied us constantly, took drugs and drank too much. At first we figured it was all because she had fallen in with the wrong crowd. Then, many crises later, we decided that she was a spoiled, ungrateful, rotten kid. Only after she ran away and we finally threw up our hands and got professional counseling did we realize that Val was seriously depressed. If we had only realized that, we would have tried to be more supportive and get help for her sooner. But how were we to know? It's so hard."

Teenage Depression Can Be Extremely Intense

This intensity is often due to physical or hormonal changes, the developmental tasks of adolescence (which include growing away from parents), shaky self-esteem and a great need for peer acceptance coupled with a lack of social experience.

While these changes and tasks don't invariably spell crisis for the adolescent (a survey of teens by Chicago psychiatrist Dr. Daniel Offer and psychologists Eric Ostrov and Kenneth Howard revealed that 85 percent of the healthy, school-attending teenagers surveyed reported they were happy most of the time), depression is a fact of life some of the time for many teens, and for those who are troubled, the tasks and pressures of adolescence can lead to intense bouts of depression.

"I believe that all teens are depressed to some degree," says Dr. Davenport. "They are suffering a great loss. They have to lose the image of their parents as perfect in order to grow up, so many adolescents are in a mourning process and feel quite alone. This depression is also cultural. In some societies breaking away from parents is not encouraged or expected, but in this country, generally, it's considered essential."

This breaking-away process is complicated by the complex variety of skills and prolonged education often required in our high-tech society. Many teens are hungry for independence, but know that realistically speaking, full personal freedom may be years away. This realization may deepen a young person's feeling of hopelessness if he or she is caught in a difficult home situation.

The changes of adolescence bring unique pressures. "At times, adolescents are overwhelmed with physical, cognitive and emotional changes," says Dr. Brown. "Life looks like a scary and immense undertaking as they confront all the changes in feelings, life tasks and a peer-oriented social world."

In this framework of tumult and separation from parents, a teen's reactions to negative experiences—a lost love, a correction by a teacher or family problems—can be intense. All too often depressed teenagers don't have the experience to know that time heals, that there is always hope, that they can survive a crisis and perhaps even learn from it. Life is often seen in absolutes—intensifying any crisis.

Teenage Depression Is Often Minimized by Adults

Part of the problem may be due to the fact that parents, too, are going through difficult life stages.

"Usually, the teen has parents in middle age who are going through their own developmental changes, their own sense of loss, and who feel, perhaps, that they are losing just what the adolescent is gaining," Dr. Mehr points out. "So the parent may react to the adolescent with some anger, jealousy and hurt."

At this stage, it's easy to look at a teenager and say, "My God, you're young! You have your whole life ahead of you. What could you possibly have to be depressed about?"

The experience gap can also be a factor. As an adult, you have a much broader perspective and are not as likely to react so intensely to every setback, loss or stressor in your life. It's an understandable temptation to say, "You'll get over it—it's not really such a big deal. Wait until you're grown up and face *real* problems!" At times our generational chauvinism leads to invalidation of all adolescent feelings and experiences.

The late Peter McWilliams, author of a number of best-selling books, recalled during an interview for the first edition of this book that he received a lot of fan mail when his first book, a collection of his poetry written around the theme of love and loss of love, was published. At that time, McWilliams was only seventeen, a fact that was not revealed in his book jacket biography or in any publicity releases about the book. "I got all these letters from adults of all ages saying how they could really identify with my feelings and how I really touched their lives and their experiences through my poetry," he says. "But I'm afraid that if they had known I was only seventeen, the reaction would have been: 'What would *you* know about love?' or 'It was just puppy love. You'll get over it,' instead of 'I understand. I've been there, too.'"

The Acting-Out Behavior of Teenage Depression Can Have a Lifelong Impact

While adult lives can be severely affected by bouts with depression, the destructive potential of serious teenage depression is even greater, with more long-lasting aftereffects. Dropping out of high school, having and keeping a baby, getting into trouble with the law, sustaining a serious injury as the result of risk-taking behavior or stunting one's emotional growth by anesthetizing painful feelings with drugs or alcohol can have a great impact on one's future, preventing a young adult from having a full, healthy, productive life—or making it considerably more difficult to do so.

Of course, there are success stories—teens who weather a stormy, troubled adolescence and emerge as strong, resourceful, productive and happy adults. But many times it's difficult or even impossible to undo the damage that destructive choices bring and to make a new start.

For example, Norman Fleishman, director of the Population Institute in Los Angeles, laments the fact that "when a young teenage girl gets pregnant and decides to keep and raise the baby herself (as most seem to be doing these days), about 90 percent of her life script is already written for her. Freedom is curtailed just when it should be increasing. Dreams go unrealized, often forever. The young teen mother is more likely than others her age to spend a lifetime undereducated, unskilled and living in poverty."

Darryl, whose depression caused him to drop out of high school, wants to try for a second chance, but his low self-esteem holds him back. "My brother is a doctor and my two sisters both graduated from college and have great jobs," he says. "I feel like nothing, working for minimum wage in a fast-food place. I keep wanting to go back to school at night and get my high school diploma, but I'm so tired after work and I was never very good with studying. I keep telling myself, 'Next year . . . next year I'll do it for sure.' "

If a teenager has the benefit of early intervention and help in coping with his or her depression, however, the life script can be quite different.

"We're finding that adolescence can be a very useful time, and the idea of the die being cast permanently at an earlier age is in error," says Dr. Lee Robbins Gardner. "Adolescence is a time for reworking ways of coping and finding ways of reorganizing the self. Many teens who have problems in junior high, for instance, can be much more successful in high school."

These possibilities make it even more imperative that teenage depression be diagnosed and treated early. For a troubled teenager, that early intervention can be of life-changing importance.

4

Early Warning Signs

How Can You Tell If It's Depression or Simply Moody Adolescence?

As you flip through the family photo album, a child smiles back at you. With a wave of nostalgia, you remember the adorable baby, the inquisitive toddler, the curious, companionable school-age child who loved to share time, interests and activities with you, a child who was affectionate and reasonably compliant.

Now, however, if your experience parallels that of many parents today, that lovely child has become something of a stranger. It may be difficult to pinpoint when things started changing. Perhaps it was when your child stopped referring to you by name and started calling you (with a distinctive inflection) *"he"* or *"she"* (as in *"He* won't let me—of course!" or, to a friend on the phone, "I can't talk now. *She* just came into the room!").

From then on, if you're like most parents, you haven't been able to do much right as your child has attacked your lifestyle, ideals, activities and goals, becoming increasingly hard to reach, moody and given to outbursts of often inexplicable anger. When, via coaxing, cajoling or vicious threats, your teen can be persuaded to join a family outing, he or she is likely to lag sullenly behind the rest of the family, ashamed to be seen with you. Many of his or her old interests and passions have faded, and as far as you can tell, your teenager spends an inordinate amount of time doing absolutely nothing. Battles over rules, responsibilities, curfews, attitudes and opinions seem to be part of your daily life together.

And sometimes you wonder what's happening here. Is this the way it's supposed to be? Is your teenager going through normal adolescent moodiness and rebellion or is his or her behavior indicative of more serious problems? Is this just a phase?

"Maybe it's just a phase" is an expression of hope uttered by many a beleaguered parent, and in many cases it is, indeed, a phase—simply part of the adolescent's process of separating from the parents.

"Oppositional behavior is a common way of separating from parents," says Dr. Marilyn Mehr. "For example, if parents expect a lot from their kids academically, poor grades can show that the child is different. He may need to define himself in this way. Also, a lot of adolescents go through a period of disorganization due to body changes, and this can affect moods, school performance and the like. Very commonly, this *is* just a phase."

Before you face an empty nest, Dr. Lee Robbins Gardner observes, you may well experience what she calls "the battered nest."

"Kids have to make it comfortable for themselves to leave," she explains. "They need to feel that they're not leaving so much behind."

As part of the adolescent transition, then, this oppositional behavior is a temporary phase. During this time you may see a number of transient episodes of depression in your teen as he or she experiences romantic breakups, cruel remarks from classmates or other major setbacks and disappointments.

How can you tell if what you're seeing is a temporary episode or phase or if it might be serious depression? The difference is usually a matter of time, intensity of depression and the amount of deviation from the child's usual personality and behavior.

In evaluating your teen's behavior, ask yourself the following questions:

HOW FREQUENT AND INTENSE IS THIS BEHAVIOR?

When a teenager is going through a rebellious phase, there are usually moments of calm between stormy outbursts and challenges to your authority. There may be surprising moments of sweetness and cooperation and some ability to get along with various family members at least sporadically. While acting-out behavior such as withdrawal from the family, temper outbursts and experimentation with cigarettes, alcohol or marijuana or cutting classes occasionally may be manifestations of adolescent rebellion, such rebellion is usually temporary and experimental in nature.

The key word is *temporary.* If a teenager regularly cuts classes, is often drunk or stoned, is constantly angry and is unable to get along with anyone in the family, he or she may be suffering from serious depression.

HOW LONG HAS THIS BEEN GOING ON?

The acting out that teenagers do to express rebellion and some transient depression is limited in time and scope.

Normally, episodes of transient depression last no longer than a few days or a week or so. In the case of bereavement, if a parent, sibling, relative, friend or beloved pet dies, it may take up to six months for the teen to work through his grief. Generally, though, it is when depression is intense and lasts for a longer period of time—at least two weeks, but usually longer than that—that your child may be suffering from major depression.

IS THIS BEHAVIOR CHANGE DRASTIC FOR MY CHILD?

While the changes that regular teen rebellion brings seem like overnight transformations, they probably started developing over a period of time as your child began preferring to be with peers, differed with you on increasingly frequent occasions and became less involved in family activities. The changes are usually not drastic. An excellent student's grades may fall a bit in the tumult of early adolescence, but it is unlikely that he or she will fail a class.

However, it is an obvious sign of trouble when behavior changes come with little or no warning and when they are drastically out of character. When an A student refuses to go to school or starts failing classes, it may be a sign of a depressive crisis.

How Vulnerable Is My Teen to Depression?

Fourteen-year-old Lisa's behavior, lifestyle, friends and general outlook on life have changed drastically during the past few months. Her parents realize that Lisa needs help, but they aren't sure what is wrong or what kind of help she might need.

You may identify with this situation. Perhaps your child refuses to tell you what he or she is feeling and is not inclined to ask for help directly. There is often an unspoken code among teenagers: "You don't tell an adult." They may confide feelings of anger or sadness to friends, who are not equipped to help. How can you begin to identify the causes of a child's depression and get help if and when needed?

Because a great deal of adolescent depression is a reaction to a combination of stress factors, you can begin by considering the following questions. *Be alert to the fact that several "yes" answers in combination over the past year can indicate that your child is especially vulnerable to depression.*

1. Has anyone in your immediate or close extended family died during the past year?
2. Has a family pet died or been lost?
3. Has your child lost a friend through death in the past year?
4. Have you and your spouse had significant marital problems recently with an increase in the number of arguments and tensions?
5. Have you and your spouse separated or divorced in the past year?
6. If you are divorced, has your child seen a great deal of you or your spouse during the past year?
7. Has your family moved within the past twelve months?
8. Has your child changed schools this year—either due to a move or due to progressing on to junior high, high school or college?
9. Has another child in your family left home for college, marriage or independent living?
10. Has a friend or romantic interest of your teenager's moved away recently?
11. Have you or your spouse experienced serious depression in the past year or two?
12. Do you or your spouse have a drinking or drug-abuse problem?
13. Has anyone in your family had a serious illness or injury?

14. Does your teenager have a chronic illness such as diabetes or epilepsy that sometimes limits his or her participation in normal teen activities or that is a source of conflict between you and your teen?

15. Has your teen had a serious or prolonged illness in the past year?

16. Has your child sustained an injury that required curtailment of his or her normal activities?

17. Has your child experienced significant physical changes in the past year—for example, a growth spurt, breast development, voice change or the beginning of menstruation?

18. Is your child lagging behind peers (or considerably ahead of peers) in physical development and is he or she getting teased because of this?

19. Has anyone in your extended families—including parents, grandparents, siblings, aunts and uncles—ever suffered from significant depressive illness?

20. Has your family had a significant change of lifestyle recently, due to financial hardships, job loss or a parent reentering the job market?

21. Does your child seem to have low self-esteem, and is he or she highly self-critical?

22. Do you have high expectations of your child and find yourself extremely disappointed—showing this disappointment openly—when your child's performance falls somewhat short of these expectations?

23. Is someone in your family, especially a parent, extremely critical of this particular child? Is this teen regarded as the family misfit or seen to be the focus of a lot of family conflict?

24. Have you felt distance growing between you and your teen during the past year? Is it difficult or impossible to communicate these days?

25. Does your teen have a learning disability?

26. Are you:

    a. a permissive parent with few rules and regulations for your teenager?

    b. a strict parent, with many rules and low tolerance for conflict or disagreements? Do you hear yourself saying "Because I said so!" or "Don't you dare talk back!" quite often?

27. Do you have reason to suspect (or do you know) that your teen may be gay or lesbian?

28. Is openly expressed anger taboo in your house?
29. Do you have trouble trusting or expressing trust in your teenager?
30. Has your teen had a significant romantic breakup recently?
31. Has he or she experienced estrangement from an important friend?
32. Does it seem to you that your teenager is often the target of teasing and ridicule from peers? Does he or she feel isolated from peers?
33. Does your teen seem unusually sensitive to teasing, criticism or indifference from peers, teachers, relatives or friends?
34. Does your teenager seem to have difficulty making and keeping friends?
35. Is your child prone to either-or, black-and-white thinking, such as feeling like a failure if he or she isn't always the best at something?
36. Have you remarried, bringing a stepparent into the family, within the last two years?
37. Is your child having difficulty with a particular teacher this year? Does he or she feel picked on, intimidated or put down by this teacher and complain more than usual about difficulties at school?
38. Has your family had an addition—birth of a baby or adoption of a child, grandparents or other relatives moving in—that has increased your teen's level of household responsibilities or decreased his or her privacy?
39. Has another child in your family made significant achievements in the past year or so? Have there been any comparisons made between siblings, always in favor of the achiever?
40. Has your teenager achieved a significant goal recently—for example, graduated, won an award, made a team, perfected a skill or otherwise achieved unusual positive recognition?

5

What Are the Symptoms of Adolescent Depression?

The symptoms of adolescent depression are many and varied. They are most significant when several occur in combination. These symptoms may include the following:

Dysphoric Moods

An increase in irritability, sadness, anxiety and expressed hopelessness may indicate depression. A depressed teen may seem bored, listless, irritable and disenchanted with life in general. He or she may exhibit little interest and pleasure in the things he or she used to enjoy.

With major depression, the teen will be irritable or depressed most of the day, nearly every day, for at least two weeks. A teen with dysthymia, or chronic depression, will have an irritable or depressed mood for most of the day, more days than not, for at least one year.

Changes in Eating and Sleeping Habits

Lack of interest in food with a major or rapid weight loss is often a clue to depression. Compulsive overeating and sudden weight gain can also be danger signals. A major change in sleeping habits is also a symptom of depression. Among the sleep disorders to watch for: insomnia, early awakening that is uncharacteristic for your child, confused sleeping patterns (for example, sleeping all day and staying up all night) or sleeping too much.

A teen with the variety of depression termed "melancholic" will awaken at least two hours earlier than usual in the morning and will generally feel more depressed in the morning than later in the day.

Social Isolation

If your teenager has no friends or has lost interest in or broken ties with close friends, he or she may be immobilized by depression. Social contact and the effort involved in maintaining close friendships might have become too difficult, or perhaps your child's friends have deserted him or her. This can be a valuable clue, since peers even more readily than parents sense when something is seriously the matter.

"Peers serve many crucial functions in adolescence," says Dr. Lee Robbins Gardner. "Teenagers need to talk with each other, to feel that they are part of a group. They use peers to flesh out their own identity and to try themselves out within the peer group. However, the dependency needs of the troubled adolescent may be so intense that others feel threatened and reject the adolescent, isolating him further."

Sudden Change in Behavior

If an A student suddenly starts failing or regularly skipping classes; if a quiet, cooperative son or daughter is suddenly belligerent, angry and taking uncharacteristic risks; if a teen with passionate interests suddenly loses all motivation, inclination and momentum to pursue them, depression could be the cause. While behavior usually changes somewhat during adolescence, the developmental changes (including oppositional behavior) are more gradual, less intense and more intermittent than the behavioral changes of depressed teenagers.

Acting-Out Behavior

Conflicts at home, running away, cutting classes, becoming sexually active, shoplifting or drug abuse—all, especially in combination, can indicate serious depression.

"Acting-out behavior is often a response to the discomfort a teenager feels, a discomfort he or she may be unable to identify or cope with," says Dr. Richard MacKenzie. "When I was in medical school, it was said that when a teenage girl was depressed, she got sexually active, and when a teenage boy was depressed, he stole cars. Now we know so much more about the symptoms and signs of depression. I believe that *any* kind of behavior that is unusual for your child should be thought of as possible depression until proven otherwise."

Hyperactivity

Many adolescents signal their distress by hyperactivity. They pace restlessly; get overinvolved in a frenzy of activities; act up in class; are nervous, anxious and irritable and find themselves unable to relax.

This hyperactivity is quite common in depressed adolescents. It is considered by a number of mental-health professionals to be a phobic reaction against depression. The depression itself remains, though masked, just under the surface.

Extreme Passivity

Loss of interest in hobbies and other active pursuits is a common symptom of depression. Withdrawal from activities, interests and friends, sulking and lying around the house or constantly watching television are also common symptoms of depression.

"Constant TV watching is often tied in with depression," says Dr. Richard Brown. "It becomes a vicious cyclical relationship. The depressed teenager watches more TV and becomes more vegetative and thus more depressed. It's important for parents to know that excessive TV watching can be a major indication of depression."

Psychologist Marilyn Mehr sees an added link between TV watching and depression. "Quite often, extreme TV watching means that there isn't much family interaction," she says. "And this can be a factor in depression."

Excessive Self-Criticism

If your teen is suddenly extremely self-critical and considers himself a complete failure, ugly, unpopular and incompetent, even when facts show otherwise, he or she may be depressed.

"Look for inappropriate guilt," says Dr. Donald McKnew. "For example, the teen may express feelings that he or she is a failure despite excellent grades, or feel that he or she is to blame for parents' quarrels." Such self-criticism reflects low self-esteem and hopelessness, which are often associated with depression.

Psychosomatic Complaints

Rick's parents are concerned because their son has been complaining of stomach pains and seems extremely tired. Yet the family doctor can find no obvious physical reasons for Rick's symptoms.

Kara has been suffering from severe headaches lately, often missing classes and spending a lot of time sleeping. Her parents are afraid that something is seriously wrong, but medical tests have found her to be physically healthy.

In some instances symptoms like the above can signal physical disease or disorders, so a thorough examination by a physician is a sensible first step. If the exam reveals no organic disease or disorder, however, depression or some other emotional disorder may be involved.

Among the common psychosomatic symptoms often associated with depression are headaches, stomachaches, lower-back pain, increased sensitivity to aches and pains and general fatigue, a feeling of being tired regardless of how much sleep one has had.

These symptoms, particularly if frequent and disruptive of a teenager's normal routine of school and activities, are strong indicators that the young person is depressed.

Substance Abuse

Abuse of drugs, alcohol or other substances can be at once a symptom and a cause of depression.

Heavy and frequent use of alcohol is, in many instances, self-medication for depression, but at the same time it can deepen the problem. Sometimes use of alcohol or other substances for social reasons brings on depression in young people.

Caffeine, another commonly used substance, found in coffee, tea, colas and chocolate, can also cause physical and psychological symptoms when it is consumed in excess. Recent medical findings have identified excessive use of caffeine as a causative factor in some instances of gastrointestinal problems, anxiety, headaches and depression.

So it can be helpful to consider your teenager's substance use habits—whether you know what they are or simply suspect what they may be—in evaluating his or her possible depression.

Risk-Taking Behavior

Driving too fast, a sudden interest in risky pursuits (such as motorcycle racing), carelessness in using safety precautions and restraint, participating in a dangerous sport or activity, running away from home and engaging in unsafe sex practices are all forms of risk-taking behavior that may be a sign of depression. Especially if the onset of this behavior is sudden and quite uncharacteristic for your child, depression may be the underlying cause.

Accidents

Constant accidents—from falling to automobile or bicycle mishaps—can be due to underlying depression. "This is a form of self-destructive behavior," says Dr. Gardner. "Of course, it's an erroneous oversimplification to say that all accidents are intentional. It could be that your child is simply clumsy or that he or she is more active and thus more exposed to the possibility of accidents than most. But keep in mind that when someone is upset, poor judgment and impulsivity are often present and can make accidents more likely to happen."

School Problems

Some of the most common symptoms of depression are related to school. These include a sudden drop in grades, a loss of interest and motivation in studies or school activities and social events, fights with teachers and classmates and habitual truancy.

Acting out in the school setting may be particularly frequent because school is a primary focus and possible stress factor in a teen's life. It is also one of the most obvious calls for help. Observes Mary Ann Dan, a special-education teacher in Los Angeles, "Kids often use school as a stage and can put on quite an attention-getting act."

School is the focal point of a great deal of rebellion, since parents and teachers often have high expectations in this area. Failure to meet those expectations is noticed promptly and with great concern.

Sexual Acting Out

Increased sexual activity can be a symptom of depression. While it is noted with particular distress when it occurs in teenage girls, boys, too, can take sexual risks that indicate low self-esteem and depression.

A teen who suddenly becomes not only sexually active but also promiscuous may be engaging in a desperate attempt to deal with feelings of depression, to increase self-esteem (by feeling wanted), to achieve intimacy and, with pregnancy, to gain the love and unquestioning acceptance of another human being—a baby.

"A girl may feel important while pregnant, and needed once the baby is born," says Dr. Mehr. "Some pregnant teenage girls express the desire to have someone of their own to love them."

This illusion of unconditional love, coupled with a lack of insight into the unrelenting demands that the complete dependence of an infant brings, leads a number of teen girls to seek pregnancy—either consciously or subconsciously—through deliberate sexual activity and contraceptive carelessness. A great number of teenage pregnancies are *not* unwanted or unplanned. Some teens see parenthood as a way to recapture the joy of the childhood they are losing, as a way to be loved and important to at least one other person, or as an antidote to depression.

In an age of AIDS, disturbing new trends in sexual risk taking can stem from depression and low self-esteem. Not all teens who fail to practice safe sex (or abstinence) at a time when sex can lead to a fatal sexually transmitted disease take such risks because they feel immune to such dangers. Sexual risk taking can have an even darker side: knowing the risks and choosing to take them anyway. Some prize the love or admiration of others more than their own health and lives. Take, for example, the teen girls in Texas who have unprotected sex with HIV-infected gang members to show their "courage and commitment" to their special men and to the gang, or on a less dramatic note, the girl who allows a boy to talk her into *not* using a condom as a show of trust and love for him. And some gay adolescents, seeing AIDS all around them, may go through denial to despair. One young gay counselor, quoted recently in a *Los Angeles Times Magazine* article about young gay men who do not practice safe sex, noted that many young men ask themselves, "Do I want to be around when all my friends are dead?"

Suicidal Talk or Behavior

If your teenager talks or muses about various methods of suicide or observes, "I'd be better off dead!" the possibility of serious depression should be considered immediately. A number of people believe the myth that those who talk about suicide never attempt it. But statistics show that many suicides are in fact preceded by attempts or verbal hints and warnings.

When your teenager even hints about suicidal thoughts, it's time to pay close attention and possibly seek professional help. And if your child has made an active suicide attempt—even a halfhearted one—it should be viewed as a warning of serious depression and a cry for help. In such instances, professional help is vital. Whether your teen talks about suicide or tries to do something about these feelings, this is a symptom that should *never* be ignored.

If you have recognized any of these symptoms, particularly several in combination, your child is probably suffering from depression.

But now that you know that depression is a strong possibility, what do you do?

Part III

UNDERSTANDING AND HELPING
YOUR CHILD THROUGH
TEENAGE DEPRESSION

6

The Ideal Way to Help Your Adolescent with Teenage Depression

Ideally, intervening on your teen's behalf means being alert to the symptoms, being sensitive to your teen's feelings (particularly to changes in mood), listening, giving loving support, helping as much as you can and assisting your teen in finding outside help if such professional intervention seems necessary.

Your actions would include the following:

Communicate Your Observations and Concerns to Your Teenager

"If your teenager shows symptoms of depression, try asking him or her if she is depressed," advises Dr. Merilee Oaks, a Los Angeles psychologist. Dr. Oaks suggests several ways to show your concern verbally, such as:

"We haven't had a chance to talk much lately. You've seemed angry at times and really down at other times. And you've been crying a lot, honey. What is it? How can I help you?"

"I've seen you crying a lot lately and I'm worried. Can you tell me what it is? If you feel you can't talk to me, can we think about finding someone else to help you? I want you to know that you're not alone—no matter how alone you may be feeling. I'm here for you and I'll always love you, no matter what."

Listen Carefully to What Your Teenager Says

You get important information and clues to your child's feelings if you know how to listen. If you're a poor listener—constantly interrupting, judging and contradicting—it's likely that your child won't tell you anything, or even if he or she tries, you won't really hear his or her thoughts or feelings.

"Keep back the 'buts,' the excuses, the attacks and the judgment," says Dr. Judith Davenport. "If you're serious about expressing the sentiment 'I love you no matter what,' this is the chance to prove it—by listening to what your teenager has to say."

If you communicate your love and caring with active, nonjudgmental listening, you are really saying, "We're in this together and you have our support. We want to help you. There is hope."

Help as Much as You Can, Then Be Open to Help from Others

As a parent, you give your teenager unique and vital help by showing unconditional love and support, by offering firm guidance, by making honest attempts to communicate and by modifying the home environment to relieve, as much as possible, the negative stressors. Examining and modifying your own stress-causing behavior, such as excessive criticism, nagging, scapegoating and the like, can be an enormous help to your teenager.

"My advice in the initial stages of a teen's depression is to be supportive and wait and see," says Dr. Donald McKnew. "The depression may be self-limiting. If symptoms persist, visit your physician, school counselor or clergyperson for assistance in deciding what further help may be needed for your child."

Dr. Lee Robbins Gardner suggests discussing your situation with a mental-health professional early on. "There are no pat answers for a parent who is having problems with an acting-out, possibly depressed adolescent," she says. "Each situation is a highly individual one and it may be most useful to talk with a mental-health professional who can help your teenager understand his or her own feelings and develop better coping mechanisms."

Realizing the limitations of your ability to help your child is difficult, but important in terms of your teen's well-being.

"It may be that you can't help your child right now because he or she is going through a period of devaluing you as a way of growing toward independence," says Dr. Marilyn Mehr. "Be open to the idea of having another significant adult person step in to help. This may be a relative, minister, teacher or friend who is better able to help right now. It may be a physician or other health professional. It can be difficult for you, as a parent, to feel secure enough to accept such help. Instead of feeling hurt, angry or jealous, see these people as complementary to your child's life. They're helping your child—not replacing you."

Why the Ideal Is So Elusive

The techniques are easy to enumerate—communication, warm support, compassionate listening and openness to outside help—but difficult to implement on a day-to-day basis, especially when your child is in crisis and you are feeling so many things: love, fear, concern, anger, frustration, desperation and confusion, to name only a few.

No matter how great your concern and your commitment to help your child, you are human, too, and the ideal is often hard to achieve for the following reasons:

YOU AND YOUR TEENAGER DON'T COMMUNICATE WELL

Your caring questions may be met with silence, anger and rejection, or you may not be able to ask the questions at all. It may well be that before you begin to communicate your love and concern for your child with maximum effectiveness, some of the communication blocks between you will have to be diminished or eliminated. As we will see in Chapter 8, this can take time, effort and a great deal of patience and commitment on your part, but it is well worth your efforts. It can change your child's life.

YOUR TEENAGER'S PROBLEMS SEEM TOO COMPLICATED AND OVERWHELMING

If your teenager is having symptoms in combination—trouble at school, conflicts with friends, drinking or taking drugs or becoming sexually active in addition to wreaking havoc at home—you may be uncertain about where to begin sorting out these problems and seeking outside help. The challenge of dealing with your child's combination of problems as well as the underlying depression, and of finding the best help you can (a necessity when symptoms are serious and in combination like this), may immobilize you. If you find yourself in this situation, you can discover special help in chapters 7 through 31. These are constructive action plans for specific problem situations and ideas for finding help that will be most beneficial for your child.

YOUR NEGATIVE FEELINGS COME BETWEEN YOU AND YOUR TEENAGER

It isn't easy to live with a depressed person of any age. It is even more difficult to be the parent of a depressed teenager. You may find that before you are able to help your teenager directly, you need to help *yourself*. This is almost inevitably the best starting point.

7

Help Yourself First: Negative Feelings and How to Deal with Them

Cynthia and Steve Bachman seem to be living the American Dream. She is an award-winning educational film producer and he is a successful attorney. Despite their demanding careers, they are loving, attentive parents to their two bright, beautiful children: Rachel, seventeen, a high school senior, and Adam, thirteen, an eighth-grader. They are well traveled and affluent and live in a lovely home in the hills overlooking West Los Angeles.

But there are flashes of anguish, anger and concern in Cynthia's eyes as she lingers over coffee, talking about Rachel. Rachel's problems have become the focus of family concerns and conflicts over the past few years.

"Our worries over Rachel go back quite a few years actually," Cynthia says, lighting her fifth cigarette in ten minutes. "When she was in grade school, she developed cancer and had over three years of radiation and chemotherapy before being given a clean bill of health at the age of ten. It was about that time—when she was ten or eleven—that I noticed her compulsiveness about cleanliness and the fact that she seemed to have trouble relating to people. I took her to a psychologist and he told me she was fine, that I should be proud to have such a bright, achieving child."

Cynthia admits that it was tempting to believe the optimistic diagnosis despite her nagging doubts. For a time it seemed to be justified. Rachel kept on achieving and not making waves for the next few years. It wasn't until her family moved from New York to Los Angeles, when Rachel was sixteen, that more obvious problems began to surface.

"The move was quite a change for Rachel," Cynthia recalls. "She transferred from her small private school to a large public school with twenty-three hundred students. She got into the honors classes, worked hard and got all A's her first semester there. She also made an effort to make friends and joined a temple youth group. But something didn't seem right with her. Then, just before semester exams, she had a sort of crack-up. She got hysterical and started screaming. I tried to talk with her and comfort her but nothing helped. I didn't realize that she was in a serious depression. She seemed better the next day and so I let it go."

Rachel's apparent recovery was destined to be brief, however.

"The real trouble came a few months later," Cynthia says, lighting yet another cigarette. "Suddenly she didn't want to go to school, started dressing in a random and sloppy way and was unable to make decisions of any kind. She was deeply depressed, complaining about her lack of friends, yet she was doing a good job of alienating the friends she did have. Our moment of truth came when her math teacher called to say that Rachel was not doing well and seemed disturbed. Soon after that, at a parents' open house at her school, all of her teachers mentioned that something seemed to be very wrong with Rachel. I immediately sought professional help for her after that."

This point in the story, rather than being a quick, happy ending, was only the beginning of the family's trials, despite the fact that Rachel's psychiatrist is one of the best in the area, that Rachel is responding well to therapy and that her family is cooperating fully in ongoing treatment.

"Rachel's depression has been harder for us to cope with than her cancer, as strange as that may sound," Cynthia says. "This is because it involves all the intricate family relationships and has such an uncertain prognosis. We have no idea when or if she might really start feeling better. With her cancer, we knew that after a chemotherapy treatment on Wednesday, she would feel better on Friday. And then, too, her surgeon had been careful to say, 'Don't feel guilty about Rachel's illness. There is no genetic link, no link with lack of care. It just happened.' Depression is another story, though When your child is depressed, you *do* feel guilty and no one can tell you any different. You keep wondering, 'Where did we go wrong? Where was the turning point? How did *I* contribute to this?' "

Guilt is only one of the troubling feelings that Cynthia and Steve have encountered as parents of a severely depressed teenager.

"My husband was devastated and didn't know how to handle the situation when it first became obvious," Cynthia reports. "He still can't cope with the ups and downs and irrationalities of Rachel's moods. I'm . . . so many things. I'm concerned, scared, hostile, angry and exhausted—for starters. As the parent of a depressed teenager, I walk an emotional tightrope. You have to be so careful about what you say and do, what you take over and what you let go. It's so hard not to catch your child's depression as you might catch a bad cold or the flu. It's so hard to deal with the anxiety and the anger. I feel emotionally battered. My daughter seems to yo-yo me back and forth between a lot of feelings. She can be very removed at one point and then hostile and angry the next. It gets to the point where you don't know how to find your center."

Although life circumstances differ, many parents know what an emotional roller coaster living with a depressed teenager can be. Like Cynthia, you may have a number of troubling and conflicting feelings: love, anger, anxiety, grief, guilt, fear and depression. There is no sure cure, no easy way out in coping with and resolving these feelings. It's important to realize, however, that you're not alone, that these feelings are not strange or unusual and that before you can help your teenager, you must begin to understand and come to terms with your own feelings.

Admittedly this is no simple task. As Cynthia relates, these feelings come in combination and are difficult to isolate. And there are no simple one-two-three solutions to what's troubling you—and your depressed teenager. But that fact should not be grounds for pessimism.

"It's important to recognize the fact that for every difficult problem, there is usually a simple solution that is wrong," Dr. Lee Robbins Gardner points out. This means, in part, that you should take time to explore your feelings and the active alternatives you may have, sorting out your situation and considering constructive coping ideas. The following are some common feelings reported in parents of depressed teenagers.

Denial

Bonnie Salazar is divorced, in her late thirties and the mother of an obviously troubled fourteen-year-old. Her son's problems are obvious, that is, to everyone but his mother. When a school counselor called her at work to say that Joe had had a number of unexcused absences in the past few weeks, that he was failing three classes and getting into fights when he did come to school, Bonnie shrugged it off as "just a phase." Later, when she discovered drug paraphernalia in their home, Bonnie readily believed her son's story that he was just keeping the stuff for a friend.

"My son and I are very close and I know he isn't a bad person," she says. "I think people overreact to a lot of teenage phases. Sure, he's having problems at school and I feel bad about it, but I really believe it will pass. Joe knows he's free to come talk to me at any time if anything is *really* bothering him."

Bonnie's denial of her son's combination of symptoms is a common and understandable occurrence among parents of troubled teens. Denial, after all, functions as a self-protective emotional reflex when a person is faced with the unthinkable and the unbearable. It is the initial coping mechanism in the face of disaster. ("This isn't happening. Not really. Not to *me!*") We may deny any of a number of things—including the harsh realities of death, serious illness and psychological and family problems. When the troubled person is your child, denial is a particularly common reaction.

WHY PARENTS DENY

Why do parents so often deny problems in their children?

Quite often the problem hits too close to home emotionally. Rod Casey was quick to deny real problems in his fifteen-year-old son's truancy, shoplifting and vandalism because he, too, had been what he calls "a wild teenager."

"I was also a very troubled teenager and needed help, which I didn't get until years later," he says. "I've spent my life being hounded by depression. It's very hard for me to see my son suffering from the same thing. As a parent, you always want things to be better for your kids. I feel guilty that maybe I've passed this depression on to my son—by acting depressed or by some sort of genetic thing. I had to get professional help myself before I could face the fact that Terry had real emotional problems."

Some parents are frightened by their teen's depression or feel like failures because their children are depressed.

"So many parents feel that the teen's problems reflect negatively on them, on their qualifications to be parents and on the family in general," says Dr. Richard MacKenzie. "Often we need to reassure parents that they are really good people who have weathered a lot of storms."

Many parents deny their children's problems on the premise that this, too, shall pass. Or they attribute problems to a simpler identifiable cause. Perhaps, they feel, a checkup or a mental-health professional holds the key to an easy and complete solution, fixing the problem child and thus transforming the troubled family scenario as if by magic.

"Quite often there are obvious problems in the whole family and the teenager is simply the one who acts these problems out," says Dr. Charles Wibbelsman. "I remember one patient, a fourteen-year-old boy with fluctuating moods and mild acting-out behavior, whose mother brought him in for a physical. The mother complained to me about the boy, labeling him as the family's major problem. In this family, the father was an alcoholic who was physically and verbally abusive to his wife and son. The mother was preoccupied with her marital problems and exhausted from holding two jobs to keep things together financially after her husband had been fired for drinking on the job. The boy was pretty okay, albeit depressed over his home situation. The mother was shocked at my suggestion that family therapy might be in order. She wanted her son to have all kinds of medical tests because she was convinced that his behavior was due to low blood sugar. She didn't want to face the fact that something was terribly wrong within the family. She wanted to feel that something simple was wrong, something I could find and fix with tests and treatment."

Minimizing and misinterpreting symptoms is another form of denial.

Family counselor Shirley Lackey recalls a joint mother-daughter counseling session in which the thirteen-year-old girl said that she felt like killing herself. The mother's immediate reaction was, "See? She's trying to manipulate me!"

"While it is true that such statements can be used in a manipulative way, as a weapon and a way of saying, 'Look what you've done to me! I don't want to live!,' you simply can't dismiss a suicide threat as manipulative," she says. "Kids *do* kill themselves. If you ignore these threats, the kid may feel he or she is out on a limb and then will go ahead and commit suicide."

HOW TO GET PAST DENIAL

While facing the reality of a child's or a family's problems is extremely painful, it is the necessary first step toward resolving conflicts and issues, exploring alternatives and making the situation less overwhelming and unbearable.

"It is much more constructive to ask yourself, 'How can I help?' rather than 'How can I deny that I contributed to this in any way?'" says Dr. Marilyn Mehr.

Guilt

Guilt is an almost universal feeling among parents of troubled teenagers. Many could identify with Cheri Koppel, the mother of a depressed fifteen-year-old girl, who says that "every time I see Jenny looking angry or unhappy, which is often these days, I wonder where I went wrong. Is it because I've worked outside the home since Jenny was three? Is it because we didn't give her ballet lessons or because I wasn't a Scout leader or a Room Mother? But because I've always had to work, I haven't had time to do those things. Would things be different for her if I had spent more time with her, asked less of her, been a more nurturing mother? I almost drive myself crazy with the guilt at times. When I don't, Jenny does. She says that her problems are my fault, that I can't understand her and that I'm not like other kids' mothers. It makes me feel rotten and leaves me wondering what to do."

WHY PARENTS FEEL GUILTY

Parents are particularly vulnerable to guilt because most feel very much responsible for their children. Some, in fact, tend to regard themselves and their children as a single unit. When parent and child don't see each other as truly separate, differentiated people, one or both may feel the successes and failures of the other intensely.

"So many parents see the child as a reflection of themselves," says school psychologist Sarah Napier. "I tell them, 'You're a separate person. When a child is fifteen, you can't be responsible for all his or her choices or activities.'"

Dr. Calvin Frederick adds that "it's important to remember that a lot of things impact on teenagers besides parents. School and peers, for example, can be very important, and what parents are contributing at this point—at least in terms of time—may be relatively little. . . ."

Still, it's difficult *not* to feel guilty when your child is in trouble, when you wonder what might have gone wrong in the teen's upbringing and how things might have been different. It is especially difficult not to feel guilty when others seem to focus all the blame on you for your child's problems.

"Too often parents are an easy target," says Dr. Frederick. "It's easy to blame parents immediately for a problem. Teenagers themselves do this a lot. But it doesn't begin to solve the problem. Both teenager and parent must take responsibility for his or her own actions."

Sometimes the lines of responsibility are difficult to discern. Sue Riley, a newly divorced mother of two (including thirteen-year-old Debbie), recently moved her family from the big, comfortable suburban home they had shared for a decade to a smaller condominium closer to the city. It meant a change of school and friends for the kids but was affordable and convenient to Sue's new job. Ten-year-old Matt seemed to adjust quickly, but Debbie became hostile and morose. She has been having difficulties at school, says she has no friends and constantly blames her mother for this negative turn of events.

Sue sighs as she relates the story of their almost daily battles. "We *had* to move. I *have* to work, and the divorce just couldn't be helped," she says, her eyes brimming with tears. "It's all very logical and reasonable, yet I feel I've done something terrible to my daughter by getting divorced and moving. But when she starts on me, I get so mad. I always end up saying something like 'I had to move, so shut up!' Then I feel worse than ever."

This situation is not uncommon, family counselor Shirley Lackey observes. "Keep in mind that you have a right to your own feelings and choices," she says. "You did the best you could at the time. When you feel you have a right to your own feelings, you can accept your children's negative feelings with some understanding and without being consumed by guilt."

HOW TO GET PAST GUILT

An important part of dealing with and resolving your guilt is realizing the scope and imitations of your responsibility. You are not responsible for everything that is amiss in your children's lives. If you take such responsibility, you can become immobilized, depressed and powerless, overwhelmed by guilt—and less able to help your troubled teen.

A more constructive plan of action is to examine your relationship with your teenager, trying to pinpoint things you have done right as well as ways you may have contributed to some of his or her problems. It is also useful to explore ways you have *not* contributed to the present situation.

"This self-examination can be painful, but it can also be reassuring and can bring about growth," says Dr. Frederick. "You may find that you haven't contributed as much to the problems as you initially thought. You may find yourself feeling less guilty and more able to help yourself and your child."

Marital conflicts, financial insecurities, necessary relocations and the like are inevitabilities of everyday life. You need to forgive yourself for not being perfect. No family or parent can possibly be perfect. No home situation, however troubled, is the sole source of a teenager's depression. Many factors, including inborn temperament and outside influences, also impact on your child emotionally and influence his or her choices and responses.

"I used to feel just terrible about being divorced and the single mother of a teenage son," says Gail Smith. "Every time Scott had a problem, I'd think that it was because of the divorce and the fact that he doesn't see his dad that much or that I wasn't doing enough. Then I started looking around and saw that some of my married friends were having problems with their kids, too!"

If a teenager tries to transfer all of the blame for problems to you, point out firmly that while mistakes may have been made in the past, making the best of a difficult situation and finding constructive ways to cope are part of growing toward maturity. Blaming another takes away much of one's own power to act, and heightens the sense of helplessness that contributes strongly to depression.

"Both you and your teenager must take responsibility for your own actions," says Dr. Frederick. "When I'm with a teenager who is complaining endlessly about a parent and blaming him or her for all existing problems, I say, in effect, 'Okay, you've convinced me that your parent is a real s.o.b. Now what?' The point, of course, isn't whether the parent really is or isn't an s.o.b., but the fact that the teenager must take responsibility for his or her own life, to go on to set his or her own house in order."

Families Anonymous, a nationwide organization of self-help groups for parents with problem teenagers, encourages members to "release with love," to let their children take an increasing amount of responsibility for the problem; encouraging their teens to cope with and learn from their own mistakes. These parents, in releasing with love, are working to avoid the trap of overwhelming guilt and a lifelong role as rescuer.

Fear

Fear has become something of a way of life for Ted and Joyce Howe. Their sixteen-year-old son, Mark, who has had diabetes for five years, has been sullen, depressed, rebellious and reckless for months. He is careless about eating on time and has started drinking occasionally with some new friends, and his diabetes is getting more and more out of control. In the past Ted and Joyce were able to control what Mark ate and keep his meals and insulin injections tied to a strict schedule. Recently, however, Mark has rejected this structured regimen. He hates feeling different from his peers and needs to deny his medical condition in order not to feel different. His parents are understandably frightened—for Mark and over their sudden loss of control.

While circumstances differ greatly from family to family, parental fears of loss of control are very common. In some instances, relinquishing some control or the notion of regaining total control of your child eases fear and tension.

HOW TO DEAL WITH FEAR AND ANXIETY

"Sometimes you get further with a teenager by giving up some control," says Dr. Marilyn Mehr. "In an instance like Mark's, it is important to put the responsibility for both treatment and control of the diabetes on Mark and his doctor so that the disease is no longer an issue between the teenager and the parents."

While stepping back and allowing your teenager to take more control and responsibility for his own life can be scary initially, it pays off by defusing the impact of rebellion in a certain area of the teen's life.

If you find yourself nose-to-nose with your adolescent over all issues—major and minor—you are helping to create a situation that erodes your ability to take control when you must. Save your fights for the major issues.

Beverly Sanders, the mother of a depressed fifteen-year-old daughter with a spotty attendance record at school, has a history of battling Suzi over school, her mode of dress and her friends. When Beverly decided to confine her rules and confrontations to her daughter's school attendance and resolved that as long as Suzi went to school she would not nag her about her manner of dressing, the tension eased. Letting go of control in minor ways while providing firm guidelines over major issues can reduce your fears and increase your effectiveness as a parent.

Firm guidelines on issues that truly matter and equally firm insistence on the teen's responsibility for making decisions in other areas help reduce fears and conflicts.

A number of parents, quite understandably, are fearful over the possible consequences of their children's acting-out behavior, which can be life-changing, even life-threatening. There are no easy answers for reducing these fears and no easy solutions to these situations. Communicating concern, insisting that the teenager try some type of professional help and, perhaps, seeking professional help for the entire family are steps in the right direction.

Vulnerability

When a teenager is wreaking havoc on their lives and their emotions, many parents feel extremely vulnerable yet fearful of letting the teenager know how his or her acting out is affecting them.

"Many parents have a need to be seen as perfect," says Dr. Judith Davenport. "They don't want their kids to see their vulnerability. But it may help to let your teens know they can affect you, even hurt you. When you express your vulnerability and feelings, your child may allow his or her own feelings to surface in less hurtful ways. I use my own reactions a great deal when I work with teenagers. I let them know how they affect me."

Sharing vulnerability can be the start of a new and better level of communication between you and your teenager. Being able to express both positive and negative feelings will defuse tension and may decrease the teen's need to act out feelings rather than simply express them.

Anger

Cynthia Bachman, whose story about her depressed daughter, Rachel, began this chapter, has become well acquainted with feelings of anger and frustration during the past year. "I've felt terrible anger and hostility toward Rachel during this time," she says. "It probably sounds terrible, saying that I'm angry with a girl who is so troubled and who needs so much help. But I am and I don't think I'm at all unusual. I sometimes get furious when Rachel acts like a five-year-old even though I know why she acts that way. I'm angry at the way this has disrupted all our lives and how long it has been going on."

Cynthia's feelings parallel those of a number of beleaguered parents. When you have a child in trouble, you worry. But you also feel very angry about the situation in general and, at times, at the troubled child.

WHY PARENTS FEEL ANGRY

This anger is triggered by a combination of factors. You see your teenager, poised on the threshold of so many choices and so many opportunities, ignoring, canceling out or not realizing his or her good fortune—and you feel angry. You may have invested many of your hopes, dreams and feelings of self-worth into your child and feel furious when he or she doesn't come through as expected. You may feel victimized, your life invaded. You are likely to feel frustrated when, even with your own and outside efforts and intervention, the situation shows no signs of quick change or resolution.

Many parents feel guilty about this anger and try to repress these feelings they consider unacceptable. But anger is inevitable. The question is how to deal with it.

THE DANGERS OF UNEXPRESSED ANGER

The problem is, of course, that unexpressed anger doesn't simply go away. It comes back to haunt us in a number of ways.

Joy and Ken Jones, frustrated and furious over problems with their son Rick, have displaced their anger onto each other, with resulting marital conflicts.

Joan Peters, a single working mother, traces some on-the-job difficulties back to her anger and frustration over her troubled thirteen-year-old son Larry. "I'm an office manager and try to be fair," she says. "But lately I haven't been succeeding too well. I've been so upset over Larry that I find myself short-tempered with some of the people I supervise, over the smallest things and sometimes without real cause."

Repressed anger can take its toll in physical ways as well. Sally McFarlane, a single mother whose fourteen-year-old daughter is seriously depressed, has been having more migraine headaches than usual during the past few months and feels exhausted much of the time. There are times when she fears that she is "catching" her daughter's depression—a real possibility.

Denying or repressing a major emotion that is stifling your feelings can become a way of life. When you repress negative feelings, you may also repress all feelings—including love, joy and happiness—as you numb yourself.

Losing your feelings can mean losing important coping tools. When you face a troubling situation, memories of having weathered other crises, of sharing joy, love and closeness with your child in the past, can sustain you in the present. But if you devote your energies to burying your feelings, you may bury these memories and the capacity to recapture the joy and hope you once had.

HOW TO COPE WITH ANGER

It's natural—even necessary—for you to feel angry right now. There is no quick or easy way out. But if you can get in touch with your angry feelings and use them constructively, there is hope. For anger is an opportunity, an energizer, when vented in constructive ways. It can inspire you to take action, to seek some solutions, to break the cycle of inertia into which you and your teenager may have fallen.

Try to pinpoint your angry feelings and their source. What can you do about your anger right now? Communicate your feelings to your teenager. Sharing your feelings in a constructive way will help both you and your teen to blow off steam. Explore ways to deal with conflicts and decrease your child's need to express his or her painful feelings with acting-out behavior.

"If you say, 'I feel angry when you stay out past midnight and don't even call,' and state your own limits about what you will tolerate, you are taking a step in the right direction," says Dr. Davenport. "It is more difficult to respond this way than to scream, 'You're doing this to drive me crazy!' But it is also a much more effective catalyst in changing a troublesome situation."

If you express your anger, you are giving your child the message that it's okay to feel angry and that there are better ways to express anger than by hurting oneself or others. Serving as a constructive model for your teen is crucial to building a more positive relationship.

If you can't get through to your teenager right now, expressing your anger to your spouse or to a friend, relative or counselor is also a helpful way to release your feelings and explore your alternatives for action. You might keep a diary. Testing your responses on paper first is a good way to find the most appropriate plan of action for the next challenge you face with your teenager.

Even physical exercise—particularly vigorous sports involving hitting motions (such as tennis and racquetball)—helps to reduce some of your pent-up tensions and frustration. All of this will leave you better equipped to cope with your ongoing problems.

Depression/Despair

When sixteen-year-old Tom Black's depression—signaled by drug use, falling grades, stomachaches and reckless driving—became evident, it was only the beginning of his family's trials. After some months, many crises and countless confrontations, his fourteen-year-old sister, Ann, is having severe headaches. His father, Dale, is increasingly impatient and short-tempered at home and at work, and his mother, Lucy, has slipped into a depression of her own.

"I don't see anything to look forward to, and this is the first time in my life that I can remember feeling that way," she says. "We've tried so hard to help Tom. Nothing works. He won't go see a counselor. Tom and his problems have taken over our lives. We have no free time, no fun, no relaxation. We've stopped entertaining and seeing friends, and Dale and I never go out anymore. It's very hard not to resent Tom for that. After all these months of trying to handle my own feelings and Tom, too, I don't have any energy left. It's terribly discouraging to try so hard and accomplish so little."

Unfortunately, Lucy Black's plight is quite common among parents of depressed teenagers. Some experts estimate that if you live with a depressed person, your own chances of developing depression may be as high as 80 percent.

WHY DEPRESSION CAN BE CONTAGIOUS

Depression tends to strike parents who are most concerned about their depressed child, parents who want very much to do the right thing, to take the best possible care of the troubled teen.

The problem is that extending such care and concern is often an exhausting, ungratifying endurance test, at least initially. The depressed teenager is not likely to thank you for your help and may even actively resent it. He or she may try to block your efforts at communication, may continue to blame you for his or her pain, may refuse helpful alternatives and may remain generally unresponsive to your sacrifices, love and pain.

Under such circumstances, it would be a bit unusual if you didn't feel flashes of resentment, anger, exhaustion and despair—feelings you might push aside because your energies are focused on helping your child. When you're under such constant pressure with no immediate happy ending in sight and myriad buried feelings depression often results. In some ways, then, depression can be catching. Unfortunately, it can become a constantly reinforced cycle of despair, impairing the quality of your life, your marriage and your ability to be an effective, loving parent.

HOW TO PREVENT OR COPE WITH YOUR OWN DEPRESSION

The key to preventing or combating your own depression is self-care. When you have a troubled teenager, it is common to become so focused on him or her that you lose sight of your own needs. But taking good care of yourself is a vital part of being an effective helper. How can you begin to take better care of yourself? The following suggestions are just a few ideas:

Keep your own life and routines as normal as possible. Resist the temptation to stop seeing friends, cancel vacation plans or drop hobbies and other pursuits you enjoy, particularly if you feel yourself slipping into depression. These pursuits can be uplifting and energizing. Get out of the house regularly—and away from the problem situation. Give yourself opportunities to step back, blow off steam, pleasantly distract yourself and seek some necessary relaxation, and support. Keeping to regular routines as much as possible will give some semblance of order and normality in your life, even in the midst of a crisis.

In spite of their daughter's problems, Linda and Steve Harrison keep to their long-established routine of Sunday afternoons alone together—browsing through bookstores, taking leisurely drives or enjoying a brunch for two. "We found that we couldn't sit worrying about our daughter every day, all day, without getting depressed ourselves," says Linda. "We give her a lot of time and care, but we need time for us, too. So Sunday afternoons are ours, and these give us a chance to relax, to get back in touch with each other, share feelings and regroup our strength and our forces for the week ahead."

Develop a support system and use it. This is especially important for single parents who may be coping, virtually alone, with a troubled teen. But it applies to all parents. If you don't have friends, family, a church or synagogue—whatever would constitute a support system for you—start building one little by little. You need support for the constant stress and responsibility you face. Enlist the aid of others you trust. Don't be shy about seeking them out. Most people enjoy being needed—and you can reciprocate by being a good friend to your good friends!

It is important, too, to encourage any constructive support systems your teen develops. Involvement with a youth group, church activities, time with friends or sharing confidences with another adult—a favorite teacher, relative, youth worker, counselor, neighbor or family friend—may help your teenager tremendously and take some of the pressure off you. But accepting such help is not always easy.

"One of the hardest tasks of parenthood is to let go and allow your child to develop intimate relationships elsewhere," says Dr. Judith Davenport. "But in order to grow up, a child must do this. It helps if you both have other meaningful people and activities in your lives."

Other significant people in your child's life will never replace you, but will help your teen grow in ways he or she must. They ultimately help to improve the quality of your own relationship with each other by helping your child's personal growth and development of new insights.

Having a united and mutually supportive relationship with your child's other parent—whether or not you are presently married—is crucial. If you can take turns coping with your depressed teen, being unified in the crisis without blaming each other or allowing your teenager to play one of you against the other, this can go a long way toward reducing some of the stresses you face daily.

"My ex-husband and I spent years hating each other," says Barbara Carroll, the mother of seventeen-year-old Amy, who was recently hospitalized after a suicide attempt. "But he has really stood by me in this. I can see how much he loves Amy, and that means a lot. And I'll never forget how gentle he was when I cried and started blaming myself for her problems after she was hospitalized. He took my hand and said, 'You did the best you could. I know you did. And so did I. Who knows why this happened. But let's work together to help Amy. We'll get through this, Barb. We'll get through it together.' That meant so very, very much. And it was a turning point—for us and for Amy."

Do good things for yourself. Taking good care of yourself means taking time out to do whatever you need to do to stay healthy, fit and reasonably satisfied with life in general. This means eating well (even when you don't feel like it), getting some regular physical exercise at least three times a week (this can be a great stress reducer, whether you take long walks, run, swim, play tennis or bicycle) and making space in your life for things you enjoy. This might mean dinner out with your spouse or a friend, involvement in a worthy cause, a solitary afternoon or a long, hot, uninterrupted bath. Particularly when you're under pressure, you need all the healthy habits, events to anticipate and satisfying or comforting outside pursuits you can get!

Restructure your priorities. Make an effort to sort out what is a crisis in your life and what isn't. Then let the less important issues go to give yourself more time and strength to deal with what really matters.

Resolve to take each day as it comes so you don't put added stress on yourself by agonizing over the past or dreading the future. When you're in the midst of a crisis, getting through each day—one at a time—is a manageable goal. Your current situation realistically is something that will probably not be resolved quickly or easily. Don't subject yourself to the added strain of expecting instant results from counseling or therapy or your own efforts to help. Major problems generally take some time to develop *and* to resolve.

Make use of professional help when you need it. Many people who need help from a psychologist, psychiatrist, marriage and family counselor or other mental-health professional avoid seeking such help out of shame. It is no disgrace to need a helping hand, but it *is* a shame to suffer needlessly or longer than necessary because you're too afraid or embarrassed to seek professional help. (See Chapter 30 for information on types of help available.) Professional counseling may involve your entire family, your teen, you and your spouse or you as an individual. Even if your teenager or your spouse refuses to seek help, don't hesitate to look for it yourself if you're having trouble finding your way out of the present crisis on your own. Seeking and making good use of professional help will do a great deal for you and your family. It will give you support, relief, new insights and added strength, and it will help to rebuild your self-esteem and hope that life will be better.

Be gentle with yourself. It is tempting—but ultimately hurtful—to be extremely self-critical when you face a family crisis. Resist the temptation and be gentle with yourself instead. You deserve gentleness. You *need* it during this time. No one is Superparent—*always* patient, understanding, compassionate, strong, wise and nurturing. Learn to let go of the need to be perfect. Even when you fall short of a goal or make a mistake, remind yourself that you did the best you could.

Learning to be gentle with yourself, to make time for yourself and your own needs is vital. You must be your own nurturing parent in order to be the person—and the parent—you want to be. You will be more in touch with your feelings and better able to communicate your concern and your love to your child.

8

Barriers That Block Family Communication

It's hard to say when the sullen silences and the angry confrontations began for Julie Frashier and her parents. Julie's early years had been tranquil enough. She had always been quiet and cooperative, and she never talked back to her parents. In the past two years, however, there has been a change.

"It started the summer she was thirteen," Sheila Frashier remembers. "She started defying us, crying a lot, arguing about everything and became highly sensitive to any criticism. She is moody and withdrawn these days. I don't know what she's thinking. I have no idea what her goals are or *if* she has any goals for now or the future."

"We never talk but to yell at each other," Don Frashier observes.

And Julie later confides that "every time my parents talk to me, it's to criticize. They don't like anything I do. I'm never good enough. In between fights, we don't have much to say to each other. I'd say we don't know each other at all anymore. They're my parents, but they don't know *anything* about who I am."

Many parents and teenagers are strangers to each other. They hide feelings and endure long silences punctuated by misunderstandings, angry words, mounting frustration and more silences. The communication gap between generations is so common that it has become something of a cliché, and it is particularly common when a teenager suffers from depression.

Why do so many parents and teenagers fail to communicate?

One factor is developmental: A major passage of adolescence is separation from parents, developing a separate, individual point of view and becoming close to others outside the family. Teens feel pressure not only to please their parents and themselves, but also to please their friends, who are now so important in their lives. It can be a tough balancing act with many painful conflicts.

Parents and teens who enjoy open communication have a better chance to compromise and agree on how much freedom and responsibility the young person can assume at any given time. But those with a history of minimal communication and poor communication skills are at a distinct disadvantage during this trying time of upheaval and conflict. These are the families of strangers who argue to no avail, who experience crisis after crisis with no resolution. Family members are caught in a perpetual no-win situation. Low self-esteem and poor communication become a self-perpetuating way of life.

Many families fall somewhere in the middle of all this. They're able to share some good times together. They find themselves able to agree or compromise in some cases, but are unable to resolve major conflicts in a satisfying, constructive way. They have trouble showing vulnerability and sharing thoughts and feelings openly.

Both teens and parents in this type of family feel some sadness, anger and regret over the fact that they seem to be losing touch. But they lack skills to break the barriers that have grown between them. Communication blocks and barriers are practically universal and incredibly varied. You and your teenager may be caught in a communication-blocking cycle in which philosophies, habits and the words you use keep you from really hearing and getting through to each other.

Communication-Blocking Philosophies

There are two common viewpoints that block communication between teenagers and their parents: generational chauvinism and the concept of parental ownership of children.

GENERATIONAL CHAUVINISM

This destructive philosophy afflicts both parents and teenagers. What it means is that each generation is convinced that the other, whether older or younger, has little of value to offer in terms of wisdom, wit or companionship.

This philosophy is fueled by the media and fashion industries, which tend to perpetuate worship of youth while minimizing teenagers *and* their elders, instead of portraying them as people with a wide variety of thoughts, beliefs and needs.

Generational chauvinists are inclined to make sweeping generalizations such as:

"What does she know? She's just a kid!"

or

"Older people think they know everything, but they are *so* out of it! Really embarrassing!"

or

"Kids today are totally irresponsible. Now, when *I* was young . . ."

or

"Adults don't know how to have fun. They never did. They were *born* dull and boring. I don't think they were ever really young."

or

"Kids shouldn't even be *thinking* about sex!"

or

"Sex? My parents???? Are you trying to gross me out, or what?"

Both teens and adults who embrace generational chauvinism feel that they have all the answers for life in general and the other generation in particular, if the other only had the brains to listen. But because each cancels out the other's credibility, nobody listens and communication is blocked.

PARENTAL OWNERSHIP

Just as common but more potentially destructive to parent-teen communication is the concept of parental ownership. Many parents feel that they should have total control over their children's lives and choices. They feel that children should accept and embrace all their values, wishes, goals and dreams. In conflicts, these parents use power rather than reason and are intent on winning. They seem to "win" consistently, especially when their children are small. However, when the children reach their teens and begin to grow physically and put more emphasis on the opinions and values of their peers, parental power diminishes somewhat. Lacking other skills to work through problems, such families find themselves locked into a continuing round of disputes and disappointments. The parents see their children as rebellious, ungrateful and unruly. The teens see their parents as tyrannical and uncaring. Neither side listens to the other, and communication is impossible.

This is a time when parents need to value each other and their children as separate and treasured people, taking pleasure in one another's competence. If you don't value your child's separateness, there can be no validation of him or her. "There are silences when there should be compliments, teasing when there should be encouragement and crossed arms when there should be reaching out," observes Los Angeles psychiatrist Dr. Saul Brown.

Dr. Brown's comments describe quite accurately the home situation of Sherry Newman, fifteen, and her brother, John, thirteen. Both have been seeing a family counselor for depression since their parents became concerned over a variety of changes. John was sleeping too much. Sherry was crying a lot. Both had little energy, were falling behind in school and seemed unable or unwilling to tell their parents what was wrong.

As their counseling progressed, it became clear that Mr. and Mrs. Newman were concerned parents, determined to give their children the best possible start in life. They were so alarmed about the prevalence of drugs, alcohol abuse, premarital sex and, as Mr. Newman puts it, "general teenage shiftlessness" in their community that they had forbidden their children to socialize with friends after school or on weekends. They were not allowed to date or go to parties. In an effort to instill a sense of pride and the value of hard work, Mr. Newman insisted that his children not only take over many household chores, but also work part-time for their ten-dollar-a-week allowances in his manufacturer's representative business. Despite their good intentions, the Newmans have alienated their depressed children.

"We don't have any time to ourselves," John complains. "Dad will give me a list of things to do on a Saturday and say, 'When you finish all that, come to me and I'll give you another list of things to do.' I never get a chance to decide what *I* want to do. I never get to do *anything* I want to do. Sometimes I feel like running away or sleeping for a week. You can't talk to my parents about this either or they think you're being a smart mouth."

"It's like what we want for ourselves or what we think doesn't count at all," Sherry says. "I've stopped trying to talk with my parents because they never listen anyway. We're hoping things will change now that we're all seeing a counselor, but so far not much has."

While the Newmans have carried the idea of parental control to an extreme, misuse of power is present to lesser degrees in many other families. In such instances there is little discussion over issues and no room for teenagers to make decisions or choices on their own (at least not without risking considerable conflict with their parents) and the question "Why?" is often answered with "Because I said so!"

As a result of their lack of autonomy or the lack of parental approval when they do show signs of growing competence and independence, the teenagers lose hope that trying to communicate with their parents will accomplish anything constructive. They also begin to question their ability to cope with life and to make independent decisions. Deprived of the pride that constructive coping and decision making bring, these teenagers tend to have low self-esteem.

It is necessary for the sake of a child's healthy development to let go gradually as he or she grows, to give him or her the power to make decisions about some aspects of life and a voice in deciding major issues. It is also vital to recognize and accept your teenager's separateness.

"It may be difficult to accept this separateness," says Dr. Richard MacKenzie. "But there are parts of your nearly grown child that you don't know anymore—aspects of him or her that you may *never* know."

Dr. Judith Davenport says that she often hears parents lamenting the fact that while they used to be so close to their children, things have changed now that these children are adolescents. And they're wondering what went wrong.

"I often reply, 'What makes you think that something is wrong?'" she says. "Growing apart, sharing closeness with others outside one's immediate family and becoming one's own person are an important part of growing up."

As a parent, you watch your child grow away from the moment he or she takes his first step, acquires the skills to feed and dress himself and learns to say no. Adolescence is simply another series of steps along the way to adulthood and full independence. Throughout this time of growth and learning, parents must keep a delicate balance between firm guidance and loving encouragement. It is painful to see your child grow away, although you feel pride and a sense of accomplishment in this growth. A parent's ability to love, to guide and then to let go gradually as the child's competence increases is essential to his growth and to good parent-teen communication.

When a parent clings too tightly, wields power too heavily, focuses on winning a battle rather than resolving differences with mutual respect and consideration, power and control become the major household issues, causing rebellion, resentment and added stress for all, as well as blocking communication.

If you find yourself in this position on occasion—unwilling to listen, to discuss differences constructively, to compromise and to let go, even in little ways—remember that while you helped to create your child's life, he or she owns it and must live it. Kahlil Gibran expressed this concept in his famous essay "On Children" in *The Prophet:*

> *Your children are not your children.*
> *They are the sons and daughters of Life's longing for itself.*
> *They come through you but not from you,*
> *And though they are with you yet they belong not to you.*
> *You may give them your love but not your thoughts,*
> *For they have their own thoughts. . . .*
> *You may strive to be like them, but seek not to make them like you.*
> *For life goes not backward nor tarries with yesterday.*

Letting go, of course, does not mean ceasing to care or to be an important part of each other's lives. In a very real sense, it can allow you to become close to your teenager in a new way, communicating more openly and effectively than ever before.

Communication-Blocking Habits

What follows are some of the more common communication-blocking habits that occur among parents. These habits become a special problem when children reach adolescence, and they also hinder your ability to help a teenager in distress.

LABELING AND BELITTLING

When problems develop, putting a "label" on your teenager can be a big temptation. It seems to be a way to pinpoint what is wrong so that the teenager can see it and change. It can also be a way for the parent to get some distance and deny any responsibility for the problem. A parent might say something like:

> "You're just a spoiled brat! That's your basic problem!"
> "You're very immature."
> "You don't know what you're talking about."
> "You've always been the problem in this family. If it weren't for you . . ."
> "You're a disappointment. . . ."
> "Why do you say and do such dumb things? You make your own problems, you know."
> "You always put your foot in your mouth, don't you?"

This approach obviously erodes a teen's self-esteem and destroys the motivation and ability to make changes. It disclaims any parental responsibility for contributing to the problem and cancels out any chance that the parent will try to help the situation by modifying his or her own behavior in any way. Above all, it destroys the trust and confidence a teenager needs to be open with a parent.

"I went through a time of feeling very alone last year," says sixteen-year-old Monica Blake. "My parents were so caught up in their own friends and activities, and things weren't going well for me at school. I started getting down on myself and really felt like I needed to be close to someone. Finally I met this guy who listened to me and really seemed to care. He helped me a lot, but my parents kept criticizing him because of his hair and the way he dressed. I tried to share my good feelings and tell Mom how much Joe had helped me find myself and she went, 'Oh, what does *he* know about anything? You're both just kids. I wish you'd see less of him. You're getting too close.'"

A few months later, after Monica's mother found birth control pills in Monica's purse, there was an emotion-filled showdown.

"I had only just started taking them and Joe and I had had sex only a few times," Monica says. "He was the first and, to this day, the *only* guy I've had sex with. But to hear my parents, you'd never know that! They screamed and yelled and called me a tramp, a slut and a lot of other names, plus I got grounded for six months and forbidden to see Joe ever again—or so *they* say. I tried to tell them how Joe and I got close in the first place and how I felt like I needed someone to talk with and be important to, but they were too busy yelling to listen. They'd say things like 'Don't talk back!' or 'Don't try to pin the blame on us!' They acted like I was taking on every guy at school. It made me feel like I can't talk to them at all because they don't care about who I really am."

If Monica's parents had been willing to listen and to *share* feelings with their daughter, they could have communicated their displeasure and disappointment over her behavior and might also have learned something important about their daughter and themselves. By labeling Monica in such a hurtful way, they may have lost the chance to be close to her.

Not all labeling and belittling is so obvious, but even in less dramatic circumstances, it can erode both self-esteem and communication.

Often communication blocks are not due to premeditated cruelty but to hurtful habits developed within the family. In many instances such habits create serious problems.

"There was a study done a few years ago comparing communication patterns in a dozen two-child families, each with one female teenager," says Dr. Alan Berman, professor of psychology at American University and a partner with the Washington Psychological Center. "Six of these teenage girls had attempted suicide; the other six had no history of suicide attempts. The families were observed conversing. In the families with suicidal teenagers, the child was constantly ignored and put down in conversations. The presumption was that this had been going on prior to the suicide attempt."

Another hurtful and belittling pattern of behavior is the "What will people think?" reaction to a teenager's problem.

Janet Zelig, for example, is fourteen and weighs well over 200 pounds. The issue of her obesity has become a major family crisis. Her slim, socially active and sports-minded parents are bewildered and humiliated by Janet's eating habits and appearance. They have begged, nagged and yelled, withheld food and marched her to a succession of diet and nutrition experts, but to no avail. Janet is unimpressed by their concern over her weight and is not willing to cooperate or to talk about her problems with them. "They're just upset about my weight because of themselves," she says bitterly. "They're just concerned about what people around here think of them, having a daughter who's overweight. They don't care about me!"

"Families get caught up in agonizing over what others will think, especially if there is the possibility that others will consider them to be bad parents," says Dr. Merilee Oaks, a clinical psychologist in private practice in Los Angeles. "The adolescent can't relate to this way of thinking. He or she gets the feeling he is being treated as an object."

These communication-blocking habits, of course, are not a parental exclusive. Teenagers fall into these themselves with comments such as:

"Nothing. Nothing's wrong. Nothing that I'd want to tell *you* about."

"Oh, *Mother,* get a life! What do *you* know about it?"

"How can I talk to you? You don't know what's happening."

"You're so unfair!"

"You're always blaming me for everything!"

"If I have to hear another one of your long, boring stories on how wonderful you all were in the sixties, I'll just die. Right here. Right now. I mean, give it a *rest!*"

In some instances, labeling and belittling are a cyclical habit—indulged in by parents and teenagers alike. They pave the way for total lack of communication.

ORDERING, PRESCRIBING AND LECTURING

As a parent, you may find yourself falling into verbal habits such as ordering ("Do it because I say so!" or "Stop feeling sorry for yourself. Just snap out of it—now!"), prescribing ("The trouble with you is that you're lazy" or "What you need is . . .") and lecturing ("What you have to understand is this . . ." or "In the sixties you wouldn't find teenagers acting this way. We were really . . ." or "Don't you know that . . . a stitch in time saves nine, Rome wasn't built in a day, and it's not wise to count your chickens before they're hatched?").

What these conversational tactics do is to communicate the idea that the teenager has no voice in decision making, that you don't trust his or her judgment, that you are not interested in anything he or she might have to say, that you the parent have all the power and that there is no room for discussion and compromise. As a result, the teenager stops trying to communicate, with the rationale that "they never listen to me anyway, so what's the use?"

The teenager stops listening, too. When he or she hears you winding up for another order, prescription, lecture or combination of the above, the adolescent is likely to tune you out and add to your frustration with eye rolls, deep sighs and expressions of long-suffering tolerance wearing thin ("Yes, *Mother!*" or "Okay, I will—*in a minute!*"). So no one gets heard, everyone feels angry and nothing is solved.

FILIBUSTERING

When some of us attempt to answer a question, make an observation or give what we feel might be helpful advice—especially if it is to our child—we unwittingly launch a filibuster that could stun a congressional veteran. It is tempting to take an idea and run with it, to give your teen all the benefits of your experience, your insights and your accumulated wisdom. The problem with such monologues, however well meant, is that they stop conversation, exasperate instead of fascinate your listener and often make your teenager less likely to seek your help and advice.

"I like to be able to ask my dad about things that bother me," says sixteen-year-old Jason Ryder. "But I figure it's not worth it if I have to sit around listening to all the stories about when *he* was my age and how well he handled everything and how he has all the answers. He does know a lot and I want to have a discussion and tell him some of the things I'm feeling, but he never gives me a chance. It's like my feelings don't matter or else he forgets I'm there."

After all, the essence of communication is sharing, so taking the floor and refusing to relinquish it for a little give-and-take is an excellent communication stopper.

TAKING OVER THE PROBLEM

When something is amiss with your child, you feel his or her hurt acutely. You may also feel a huge temptation to take over and make his problem yours. You may do this automatically without much thought.

"If I have a problem, I don't let my parents know, if I can help it," says Ron Daniels, sixteen. "My mom's usual reaction is to get all upset, even cry. The last time she cried was when I didn't make the varsity basketball team. I was feeling down and wanted to talk about it, but the way she reacted made me feel worse. I felt guilty for making her feel bad and would tell her, 'Oh well, it's okay. Don't get upset, Mom" when *I* needed to be comforted myself. My dad is worse. Tell him a problem and before you're finished talking, he has ninety-two solutions that *he* wants to act on—like 'Why don't I call and talk to the coach?' and things like that. It's just easier to talk with my friends or just figure things out on my own."

Another way of taking over a problem is by seeing it as a personal affront, as something your child does *to* you.

"When I was feeling really depressed last year and couldn't stand to go to school unless I had a drink first, I knew I was in trouble," says Diana Leonard, fourteen. "I felt like my parents had all these expectations about me being the perfect daughter. When, at the urging of my school counselor, I tried to talk with them and tell them that I was depressed and that I was scared I had a problem with alcohol, you know what their reaction was? 'How could you do this to us? We trusted you and you've let us down.' It was like I was a horrible person because I had this problem. My parents eventually got us into counseling together, but that first reaction from them hurt a lot. It didn't make me glad I confided in them—at least, not at first."

The key to avoiding this communication-blocking habit is to determine who *owns* the problem. This requires that you see your child as a separate person with his or her own life and set of problems, which may or may not be problems for you.

For example, if a teen fails to make a team, feels rejected by a friend, gets into trouble at school or feels embarrassed about a comparative lack of physical development, he or she owns the problem. Any of these will naturally be of concern to you, the parent, but when you see them as your teenager's problems, then you are in a better position to help your son or daughter cope. You will not be as likely to feel victimized or immobilized by problems that are not really your own. You will be better able to listen and to help your teen work through the problem, thus acquiring a valuable life skill. On the other hand, when you take over and try to solve your child's problems for him, he may feel loss of self-esteem, he may suspect that you don't trust his ability to come up with effective ideas and solutions on his own and he may angrily reject your advice with the accusation "You're treating me like a baby!"

If some aspect of your teen's behavior is a problem for you but not for him, it's important to make this clear. If, for example, your daughter has been coming in half an hour after curfew for the last several weeks, that extra thirty minutes out may be just fine with her, but worrisome and irritating for you. Approaching the problem in the spirit of "I get very upset and worried when you come in late" may open the door to communication—helping her to see your side of the situation.

GIVING MIXED MESSAGES

We don't always say what we mean—or mean quite what we say—and the result is confusion, misunderstandings and blocked communication.

"Some parents give subtle encouragement to their children's conflicts," says Dr. Lee Robbins Gardner. "For example, when a boy cuts school, his father might say, 'I never had the guts to do that' or 'I did that, too.'"

When such encouragement occurs, mixed with prohibitions against the behavior, it results in a great deal of confusion and conflict.

Strict and constantly repeated prohibitions also carry a mixed message. "In this way, you may subconsciously encourage a child to act out in these ways, as a way of fulfilling one's own needs," says Dr. Doris Lion, a psychotherapist in Encino, California. "For example, a parent may tell a young adolescent daughter, 'Don't you dare have sex! Don't you dare get pregnant!' On one level, the parent means this. On another, by focusing so strongly on sex, the parent is subconsciously encouraging the child to act out sexually, maybe as a way to make up for lost opportunities in the parent's own youth. It is helpful to examine your own childhood and feelings behind every very strong prohibition you voice. It's important, of course, to convey what behavior is acceptable to you and what isn't and which values you cherish and hope your child will at least respect. It may be quite another matter, however, if all your concern is focused on one area and expressed in such strongly prohibitive terms."

Subtle or not-so-subtle put-downs are also contained in some mixed messages. In many instances a parent's original intent is to encourage, and he or she may not realize how clearly negative implications ring out to the teenager.

"My personal bias is against the word 'potential,'" says Dr. Randi Gunther, a psychologist in Palos Verdes, California. "Telling a child 'You have such potential' *seems* to be encouragement, but it also means 'You're not so hot now.' It is much more constructive to focus on special qualities, abilities and talents the teenager has now that can be developed and used now and later in life."

Sandra Shelton, seventeen, says that she tunes out whenever her mother says, "You have a beautifully shaped face." Why?

"Because it's her standard introduction to her standard beauty lecture and critique," Sandra says. "What it really means is 'The shape of your face is great, but everything else about you is the pits.' It makes me feel so bad I stop listening. I know some of her advice might do me some good, but I get too hurt and mad to follow it. I feel like unless I look perfect, she won't accept me as a worthwhile person."

Saying things such as "I'll be so proud of you when you graduate from college!" communicates to your teenager that you aren't proud of him or happy for him now. And the sweetness of some successes is soured by mixed messages when the teenager tries to share the news with you. Saying things such as:

"That's nice, but don't get a big head about it."

"Second place? Why didn't you come in first?"

"Of course you did well. You're our son!"

"Oh, fantastic! Wait until I tell my friends."

can sabotage a young person's enjoyment of his achievement in a number of ways. What the above messages are really saying is: To talk about achievement shows conceit; second place is an occasion for disappointment; the achievement was nothing important, simply expected behavior; and the achievement is *yours,* not your teenager's, and your greatest joy is in sharing it with friends. In each case, the child is left feeling unappreciated and inadequate.

Another category of mixed messages comprises "yes" messages that really mean no. For example, instead of telling your teenager that he or she can't go scuba diving with a group of fairly inexperienced and unsupervised friends, you might find yourself saying, "I guess you can go if everyone else goes, but I don't think it's safe and I'll worry about you every minute you're gone. Have a good time!"

This puts the teenager in a no-win situation. If he goes, he feels guilty. If he stays home, he feels deprived. It is much more constructive to make your feelings clear—for example, "I feel that you would be taking unnecessary risks in this situation and I can't give you my permission to do this. If you and your friends took a course in scuba diving and then went out under the supervision of an experienced diver and instructor, I might change my mind. Until then, I have to say no."

Mixed messages that put your teenager down, place him or her in a no-win situation or imply that he or she is not trusted are very effective communication blocks, creating a great deal of distance between parent and teenager.

DISHONESTY

Sometimes parents say dishonest things or deny reality, hoping to encourage their teenagers. But the teen often sees the essential dishonesty and feels worse because of it.

"I saw a fifteen-year-old boy in counseling recently," says family therapist Shirley Lackey. "He was depressed over being too short and small to make the football team and was upset because his parents had been promising him he would grow—even though he was well into puberty. Being short really bothered him. It is much more constructive to help your teen explore ways to feel good about himself or herself at present—without any changes happening—and to find other interests to pursue."

Honest praise and encouragement can help a child or teenager greatly. But exaggeration and dishonesty can make the teen discount your point of view altogether. If you tell your teen that he or she is the greatest writer or singer or actor or athlete when he or she is interested in it but average or less in ability or simply still in the process of learning the skill, the teen may pick up on the difference between your judgment and reality and promptly lose faith in your opinions.

"My mother thinks every essay I write is the greatest," says Beverly Brown, fourteen. "That's nice, but when I want constructive criticism or to share something I really like, I go to Dad. When he says something is good, I know he's sincere and probably right."

Another form of dishonest noncommunication is hiding feelings and insisting that something doesn't bother you when it does, avoiding confrontations with the person directly involved in your conflicts.

"My mother has this little habit of not telling me when she's bugged about something," says fifteen-year-old Mike Saunders. "She'll act like everything is fine, then run to Dad and complain about me doing this or not doing that when she never told me it was a problem. Then Dad comes down on me like a ton of bricks and she plays the innocent martyr. It's disgusting."

Dishonesty, which can be seen as lack of understanding, trust and caring, is a highly effective communication block.

INTERROGATION

Asking too many questions can create distance and block communication, especially when you're dealing with teenagers. While it's important to ask for and have certain information, such as where your teenager is going and with whom, a barrage of questions when the teen is trying to tell you about a problem or some troubling feelings interrupts the flow of his or her thoughts, gets the conversation off on unwanted tangents and, if such questions are worded in a negative way, sets you up as a judge, making the teen less inclined to try to communicate.

Trying too hard to get your teen to open up can also have a blocking effect.

"When I get home from school, I'm tired," says Patti Reine, sixteen. "Usually it has been just another long, boring day, you know. But my mom meets me at the door almost and goes, 'What happened today? What's new and exciting? What did you do? Who did you eat lunch with? How is Spanish class coming along?' I know she's real interested in me and all, and I appreciate it to a point, but I get turned off by all her questions, especially her 'What's new and exciting?' Usually *nothing* new and exciting happens at school and that's bad enough, but when I feel Mom expects me to bring home exciting news every day, it just makes it worse. I'd like to talk more to her, but she runs at me with all these questions and I just feel like running the other way. Usually I just say, 'Nothing happened!' and run to my room and shut the door fast."

It would be more effective to create an atmosphere of warmth and openness and to keep the questions to a well-thought-out minimum.

GETTING STUCK IN THE "OLD INFORMATION" RUT

If you're like most parents, you find yourself bringing up certain observations again and again while your teenager reacts with anger and resentment and begins to tune you out. If you don't want to be tuned out, take care not to linger over and rehash information your teenager already knows. Old information sounds a lot like nagging. Statements such as "This is the third C you've made in geometry this year!" or "You're only fourteen! You're just a kid!" do not give your teen any new insights into his or her problems. Keep observations current ("You seem to be having some trouble in geometry class" or "I feel that you're not quite ready emotionally for that kind of responsibility") and focus on things that can be changed within a relatively short period of time. This will prevent some communication blocks.

DENYING YOUR CHILD HIS ADOLESCENCE

If you expect your teenage son or daughter to be a little adult and, possibly, to function as a pal, a peer and a true helpmate—and you express deep disappointment when he or she shows a lack of mature judgment or other condition congruent with adolescence—you may be setting up a communication block by denying who your teenager really is: a young person in transition to adulthood who *will* at times make mistakes, be immature or disappoint you. It isn't reasonable to expect a teenager to be a peer or a pal to you. He or she still needs a parent.

"I remember writing in my diary when I was ten that 'I know some things that kids shouldn't have to know,' " says Ashley Clark, sixteen. "I still feel that way when my mom goes on and on to me about how she hates having sex with my dad, who has diabetes and has . . . well . . . problems in bed. I guess it takes a long time or something. I don't know. I don't even want to think about it. It embarrasses me to hear stuff like that. Mom thinks we're close, but I feel very uncomfortable around her. Sometimes I get mad and feel like saying, 'Get a life! Get a friend your own age! Or see a shrink! Just don't talk to me about this anymore!' But I don't say that because I feel bad that she's unhappy and I try to be a good daughter. But it doesn't make me want to confide in her. It makes me feel like 'Oh, God, just leave me alone!' and like I'm really alone in the world. Do you know what I mean?" She suddenly looks near tears.

Appropriate boundaries are vital to good communication. If, like Ashley, your child feels intruded upon with inappropriate confidences from a parent, he will withdraw or rebel—and an important opportunity for loving communication will be missed. Keeping a clear view of which problems are appropriate to share with the family, which should be between you and your spouse and which might be best discussed with a professional therapist will help to establish these essential boundaries. No matter how mature your teenager seems, he or she is still, in many ways, a child. To blur the distinction between parent and child, teen and adult is to deny your child this essential transition period and, possibly, can cause resentment and solid communication blocks.

MINIMIZING THE SITUATION

What seems trivial to you from an adult's perspective may be a major problem for a teenager, who may feel a great need to talk about feelings of anger, loss and grief, a rejection by a friend, a broken romance, the loss of a pet or failure to reach a goal such as making a team. Such sharing will be short-circuited, however, if you try to console the teenager by saying that it doesn't matter.

"I tried to tell my dad about how crushed I was when Ben dropped me for my best girlfriend," says Jana Wiesman, thirteen. "He didn't take it seriously. He acted like it didn't matter that my world was falling apart—with no boyfriend, no best friend anymore. He just said, 'Don't worry, sweetheart. Men are like subway trains—there's another one along every few minutes. Next week you'll be in love with someone else and won't even remember Ben!' But that's not true! Getting dumped and being totally betrayed by my best friend both hurt a lot. Dad just doesn't understand."

Telling a teenager that he or she shouldn't feel a certain way also sabotages communication. Saying, "You shouldn't be so upset. It isn't that important" or "You're getting all worked up about nothing!" minimizes the problem and denies feelings that the teen is trying to share. While the teen may lack perspective, this is something he or she needs to acquire by working through his or her feelings first. Denied that chance, the teen will feel unaccepted, unheard and frustrated. It is far more constructive to say things such as "That really hurts, doesn't it?" or "I know it's really hard for you right now."

WITHDRAWING

Some parents withdraw from their children in a number of ways. They may say, clearly or subtly, "Don't bother me now," when a teenager tries to talk with them. Some listen halfheartedly—not making eye contact, reading or watching TV—with minimal response while the young person is talking or rely on the unspoken message that the teen had better not bring the parent any bad news. In these homes, it's not okay to have problems and to talk about them openly. This lack of emotional availability seriously impairs communication.

If you truly can't be available because the boss has come for dinner, you have a raging migraine, you're walking out the door and late for a crucial meeting or the issue being raised is very troubling to you and you need time to think it over, it is more constructive to make this clear to your child and set definite plans to discuss the matter later—*and then follow through!* You might say how much you want to hear the teenager out and arrange a block of time together as soon as possible. If you find yourself avoiding an issue your teen is trying to raise, telling him or her how you feel may smooth the way to communication. Saying, "I have a lot of trouble hearing about that. I have so many feelings that get in the way, but I do want to listen and to understand your point of view" is more likely to elicit favorable results than "Don't talk to me about that."

Words and Phrases That Block Communication

There are many words and certain tones of voice that quite effectively block communication with your teenager. The following are just a few of the most common ones:

"The trouble with you is . . ."
"In *my* day . . ."
"You're wrong."
"Why would you feel like *that*?"
"That's a stupid thing to say!"
"Don't you dare talk back to me!"
"You're a real disappointment to me."
"You're stupid . . . bad . . . incompetent . . . lazy . . . (etc.) . . ."
"Are you trying to drive me crazy, or what?"
"How could you do this to me?"
"Is that *all*? I thought it was something important."

"What did you expect? You're just a kid, after all."

"Don't bother me now."

What a teenager needs to tell you will not always be what you want most to hear, but in building good communication and growing past blocking habits, listening and being there for your child—no matter what—is crucial.

9

Where Does One Begin?

Why Pick on Parents?

Teenagers, like parents, block communication with their own array of habits, attitudes and phrases. They can foil our best attempts at tolerance, compassion and getting back in touch. But to focus on teenagers and the need for them to change would be self-defeating. You can change only your own feelings, habits and behavior. As you begin to relate to your teenager in a new way, your son or daughter may become more responsive to you.

Taking the first steps toward open communication may seem to be an overwhelming task. But improving communication—taken step by step and day by day—is possible and manageable. There are five major steps toward better parent-teen communication—in day-to-day living and in a crisis. These steps can be excellent preventive measures and equally excellent ways to begin to deal with your child's depression. These steps include:

1. Developing empathy for your teenager.
2. Spending time helping your teen develop survival skills.
3. Learning family stress management.
4. Staying in touch with your teen—and recognizing the healing power of hands-on parenting.
5. Creating an environment for good communication.

Empathize with Your Teen

Developing empathy for your teenager means understanding his or her point of view, seeing the world as he sees it. Despite the fact that times and circumstances of family life have changed in many ways since your own adolescence, many of the major conflicts and concerns of the teen years have remained constant. It should be helpful, then, to take a trip back in time and reexperience your own adolescence.

"Remember those times as they *really* were, not as you may have romanticized them over the years," suggests Dr. Marilyn Mehr. "You can do this a number of ways. Maybe you could start a journal where you write down memories and relive them in that way. Or perhaps you can share memories with your spouse or with a group of friends who are also parents. Ask yourselves questions about all kinds of adolescent experiences and concerns, from skin problems to romances to fears. Immerse yourself in what it was like to be an adolescent."

Some questions to ask yourself include:

• What were three of the most terrible things that happened to me when I was a teenager?
• What things embarrassed me most?
• What things did I enjoy most during those years?
• What physical problems did I worry about most?
• What is the worst thing anyone ever said to me when I was a teen?
• Who was my best friend? How much time did we spend together? What did we enjoy doing most? What special secrets did we share?
• What did it feel like to lose a friend? Change schools? Get yelled at by a teacher?
• What were my grades *really* like?
• What dreams did I have for myself? What did I want most for the future?
• What was my idea of an absolutely perfect day back then?
• Was I *really* good about helping around the house or did I ever have to be coaxed, cajoled or nagged to pitch in and do my share of chores?
• What issues sparked arguments between my parents and me?

- How well did we resolve those conflicts?
- What did my parents criticize about me or my behavior?
- What qualities in me did they praise?
- What were my honest, deep-down feelings about my parents when I was fourteen or fifteen? (You might try writing a paragraph describing your parents from your teenage perspective or hunting up an old diary if you had one.)
- How much time, from day to day or week to week, did I spend with my parents?
- How did I feel about participating in family activities versus being with my friends?
- How much did I *really* confide in my parents?

Recalling your own teenage pains, pleasures and experiences will help you to understand better what life is like today for your teenage son or daughter.

"Remembering what it was really like to get a bad grade or a reprimand from a teacher or to lose a friend, remembering your feelings, your fears and your upsets will help you to understand your teenager," says Dr. Merilee Oaks. "However, it is very counterproductive to go on and on to your teenager about what a hard time you had or, worse still, to compare your adolescence with his or hers by saying something like 'I had to live through much rougher times.' It is much better to say something like 'I know it's hard for you right now.'"

Remembering your own adolescence will also help when you're feeling shut out and rejected by your teenager.

"If your teenager is trying to separate from you and you're reacting with hurt, anger and fear and wondering, 'How is she going to cope without me telling her what to do?' just remember your own teens," says Dr. Mehr. "And ask yourself, 'How much did I *really* listen to my parents?'"

Help Your Teen to Develop Survival Skills

In order to survive the pressures and difficulties of teen life in these times, adolescents need a variety of strengths and skills. Among these are knowledge about choices and risks, social skills that enable them to be a part of their peer group and yet able to make the individual choices—such as saying no when they need to—that are optimal for them, stress management and relaxation techniques and strong self-esteem.

How can you help your teen in these ways?

• *Face the fact that teens indulge in risk-taking behavior for a variety of reasons and help your teen to find more constructive ways to cope.* You may not want to contemplate the fact that your child might deal with depression in some potentially destructive ways—drug or alcohol abuse or sex too soon— but facing facts is a necessity in order for you to have any credibility with your child and to be a real help to him or her.

Historically, there has been a major disparity between parental knowledge and teen actions. According to a Louis Harris poll for the Metropolitan Life Foundation a few years ago, 36 percent of parents surveyed said that they thought their children had tried alcohol, while 66 percent of the students polled said they had. While 17 percent of students said that they had used drugs, only 5 percent of the parents knew or guessed the truth.

So your teen, especially if depressed, can be at risk. You can help your child find more positive ways to meet his emotional needs by talking, with self-esteem-building activities or relaxation techniques, or by knowing how and when to say no.

• *Work on social skills—not only the skills to fit into his peer group, but also the skills to stand up to his peers and say no when he needs to.* A 1993 study by psychologist Antonius Cillessen of Duke University found that kids singled out for rejection by peers tended to be shy and awkward or those who were aggressive bullies. If your child falls into either category or needs honing of other social skills, helping him or her by practicing, role-playing, making suggestions and giving praise for small victories can make a major difference.

In the same way, you can help your child learn to say no.

In a study of 2,000 California schoolchildren, Dr. Linda Grossman, a psychologist in Laguna Niguel, found that preteens and teens who worked with their parents in a special program aimed at developing social and assertiveness skills were much less likely to be taking drugs three years later than those who had practiced these skills only in a classroom setting.

"Parental involvement is *the* crucial element in a child's ability to make positive decisions and say no to peer pressure," Dr. Grossman contends.

Dr. John Clabby, a psychologist at the University of Medicine and Dentistry of New Jersey, agrees. "Parents need to make a shift from trying to solve their child's problems to helping the child develop the ability to make his or her own decisions. This is crucial because you can't be there in the millions of instances when a child needs to make a decision alone in the face of peer pressure. If you can help your child feel that his ideas are worthy, he is not going to be won over by peers pressing him to do something dangerous."

Role-playing and rehearsing problem situations can help. "You might rehearse your teen being offered a cigarette or beer or a joint or facing friends who are jeering or who won't take no for an answer," says Dr. Grossman. "Together, rehearse what your child might say until his skill and confidence grow. You might also explore your child's fear of being different and what this can mean. If it means losing a friend, talk about how likely it would be to lose a friend so easily, what makes a true friend and how daring to be different can be difficult."

• *Play an active role in enhancing your teen's self-esteem.* You can do this with honest praise and interest in and validation of your teen's interests, hobbies and pursuits. It's vital to attend sports events, school plays, open houses and other events. Showing an interest in or willingness to explore some of your teen's pursuits can help your teen to grow in self-esteem and can also give you a chance to know and to help your child in many ways.

Anthony Delaney, seventeen, has had myriad difficulties during his high school years. He has been embarrassed about his dyslexia, which has made schoolwork difficult, and his self-esteem has suffered considerably as he wonders how he fits into his academically inclined family. Two years ago he and his best friend, Josh, discovered desert hiking and shared tales of their adventures with Anthony's parents, Jack and Nina. "We'd listen and ask about every detail—and his face lit up as he spoke," says Nina. "He finally asked if we'd be interested in trying a hike and we said we would. I never liked the desert before, but seeing it through his eyes, I got a new appreciation for it. It meant a lot to Tony that he could teach us and show us something—and that we were interested in learning. It made a big difference in how he saw himself and how he felt within the family. It has also given us the means to help him in a crisis.

"When his friend, Josh, was killed in a car accident last May, we had a private memorial service for him—just the three of us—out in the desert. We sat in the area where they had always camped and talked about our happy memories of this place and of Josh. We laughed with him at the funny memories and held him when he cried. And we all slept under the stars that night and felt very close. It was an important part of Tony's healing and an important event for us as a family. We wouldn't have thought to do it if we hadn't listened to this interest of his, taken time to know his friend . . . and understood how terrible this loss was for him. It made such a difference for Tony—for all of us."

Taking an interest and being there for your teen doesn't necessarily mean participating actively in all her pursuits. But knowing what she enjoys, what she does well, *noticing* what's meaningful to her and letting your teen know that you've noticed and that you admire a special talent or interest can make a major difference.

Too many parents assume that, because they are trying so hard to separate from parents and so often disagree with parents' views and advice, that parental thoughts and feelings don't matter to teens. This is not the case. Even if they don't let you know it (and even if they seem to attack everything you say), your values, opinions and commitment to your teen matter immensely.

In a recent essay contest sponsored by *The Honolulu Advertiser* for high school students, teens were asked to write about their greatest hero. All but one of the top-five finishers wrote about a parent. In several cases it was a parent who had stood lovingly and firmly beside the teen in a crisis. The fourth-place finisher, a seventeen-year-old named Heather, wrote about her nightmare with "emptiness, pain, drugs, bad grades and wishing I was dead." Her divorced parents agonized over how to help, and finally Heather's mother sent her to live with her father in Hawaii. Heather remembered getting off the plane with her eyes nearly swollen shut from crying and feeling his warmth and the security of his embrace. She wrote that her father is her personal hero and her best friend because he has been there for her in the rough times, concluding that "my hero walked into my life when the rest of the world walked out."

Being very much a part of your teen's life can make all the difference in your relationship and in your teen's self-image as he or she sees himself reflected in your eyes as someone who is very much loved and valued.

Learn to Manage Stress as a Family

Although it's optimal to keep family stressors to a minimum during the difficult periods of a child's life—for example, not getting a divorce just when a teen is starting junior high or moving just before his senior year of high school—life doesn't always cooperate.

Even in a highly stressful event, a teen can feel loved, valued and secure if the stress is handled in a constructive way by parents.

Noted pediatrician Dr. T. Berry Brazelton conducted a study some years ago to determine what best protected teens at times of major stress and risk. One of the two major protectors was a passionate interest in something. The other protective factor was being part of a family that had successfully survived a crisis, a family that had stuck together, talked and worked out a solution. He concluded that stress can't destroy a family (or a teen); it is the way it's handled that is crucial. Sharing coping strategies, talking, being emotionally available, modeling ways that your teen can find comfort or comfort himself—all of these can safeguard your teen through stressful times.

Stay in Touch with Your Teen

This means not only keeping in emotional touch, but also finding acceptable ways to give your teen physical affection. Many parents stop touching their kids when they get to be teenagers. Maybe the teens don't like being touched and kissed the way they were when they were little. Maybe the parents, noticing their budding sexual maturity, back off with caution. But human beings of all ages thrive on touch.

In fact, in a recent study at the University of Miami Medical School of seventy-two children and adolescents, half of whom were hospitalized for depression and half of whom had adjustment disorders, Dr. Tiffany Field found that regular neck and back massages were effective in reducing anxiety and depression.

Touch can be healing. It doesn't have to be a massage, if that doesn't feel appropriate. A touch on the shoulder, a squeezed hand, a quick hug, a kiss to go with verbal praise . . . all of these can help your teen feel cherished and valued.

Create an Environment for Good Communication: Questions and Exercises

Communication grows and flourishes in an environment of mutual trust and respect, which is possible only when family members feel good about themselves and each other. Begin to evaluate and make changes in your home environment by considering the following questions:

HOW DO YOU FEEL ABOUT YOURSELF?

Would you say that your own self-esteem is high, moderate or quite low? Do you accent the negative in your own life? If so, you may be passing this habit on by example to your child.

Exercise: Make a list of your good qualities and other things you like about yourself. Don't let any negative comments creep into your list. Keep it positive. Include examples of situations you handled admirably—in a social setting, at work, at home, with others or alone—in ways that were constructive and helped you to feel good about yourself, even if they occurred years ago.

For example, Penny Riordan, the mother of three teenagers, likes the fact that she is "well organized most of the time, a hard worker, a person who cares very much about my husband and children and who tries to tell them so both directly and indirectly. I'm also good at my job [computer programmer] and I am conscientious and good at keeping confidences. I also like the fact that I can be diplomatic yet honest. I've had to work at developing my assertiveness and have improved a lot. I can disagree and stand up for myself without being witchy. I can and do admit when I've made a mistake, too, which I like a *lot* about myself. I try to be sensitive to others' feelings. Sometimes I do well at this and sometimes I don't, but I'm pleased that I try to be considerate."

Take time to think about and list your strong points. It will help you to get out of the habit of accentuating your negative qualities to the point that they take over your image of yourself.

When you begin to feel better about yourself, you will have more energy and confidence to improve your relationships with others. You will also be more likely to have and to express positive feelings about your teenager.

HOW DO YOU FEEL ABOUT YOUR TEENAGER?

Do you see him or her as a trial, a burden, a mixed blessing, a difficult person, a stranger, brimming with promise or a hopeless case? How did you see this child as a baby? As a small child? Has your opinion of him or her changed drastically as he or she has grown? Some parents love and enjoy infants and small children but find little joy in sharing their lives with a teenager.

"The child in this instance can become very depressed and feel that he or she has let the parents down by growing up and becoming more independent," says Dr. Donald McKnew. "In our clinic, we see a lot of kids who feel bad about not being able to live up to parental expectations and standards."

Do you have a need for your teenager to be a certain way—for example, clean-cut, industrious, an achiever, an A student, compliant or artistically inclined—to be acceptable to you? Or are you able to accept your child as he or she basically is? Do you have a long list of complaints about your teen? Can you find anything at all to admire and enjoy about him or her?

Exercise: List qualities you like most in your teenager. If you're feeling very angry, battered by conflicts or confused and frustrated by your teen's depression, it may be difficult to come up with much at first. Keep at it. Try to think of ways your teenager has been kind, thoughtful, helpful, resourceful, brave or honest.

"When I started my list about my daughter, Lisa, I felt it was pretty hopeless," says Dan Wiley. "All I could think about was how she was driving me crazy, how insolent she could be, how hard to reach and the like. Well, the first thing that occurred to me is that she seems to be a good friend to her friends. She's loyal and giving and listens for hours to their problems, stories about boys and school and whatever else they discuss. I've noticed that she listens well when her friends visit and when she's on the phone, and that's a quality I admire. She is also very health-conscious and takes good care of herself, which is a good habit to get into at her age. She's very kind to the old woman next door, who recently lost her husband—taking her cookies, helping her with shopping from time to time and always saying hello and stopping to talk when she sees her. I know she is also trying to get along better with her little brother, who can be a pest. He goads her a lot, but she is getting much better at not rising to the bait. She's great at games—chess, backgammon, you name it. I enjoy playing those games with her because she gives me a real challenge. She comes up with some interesting ideas and I like her original turn of mind."

It's important to find things to praise in your child whether or not he is an achiever.

"All children need praise—the achiever and the less gifted child," says Dr. Richard Gardner, author of a number of excellent parenting books, including *Understanding Children: A Parent's Guide to Child Rearing.* "A gifted child should not be deprived of praise, and a parent should also encourage a less academically gifted child to find gratification from other channels. It is important to be open-minded about this. If you are open to the value of each child's individual strengths, whatever they may be, you will do all your children a great service."

It's also vital to make sure that your expectations for your son or daughter are realistic. "Realistic expectations are *so* important," says educational psychologist Sarah Napier. "Normally, a teenager can't go from a C to an A in a class in only six weeks, no matter how hard he or she works. Also, if a child is gifted, some parents expect the child to be gifted in all areas. This, again, is not realistic. In the same way, a learning-disabled child is not disabled in all areas."

Some parents also miss the importance of positive reinforcement. They are quick with criticism and stingy with praise, perhaps echoing the words of one father who said, "When my kid messes up, he needs to be told. When I criticize him, it's to help him do better. When he does well he knows it. I don't need to tell him. He *should* act that way. Why should I praise him for doing something he should do?"

Praising your child when he does something right makes such behavior rewarding to the child as well as to you. This positive reinforcement makes it more comfortable for your teen to choose these positive behaviors.

And praise from a parent who knows the child so well has a very special meaning to the teenager, even though he or she may not let on.

HOW DO YOU CRITICIZE YOUR TEENAGER?

Do you label him or her as a person, or focus on behavior? Labeling, belittling and criticizing your child's personality instead of making it clear that you love him but disapprove of his behavior can be a factor in a teen's low self-esteem, depression and noncommunication. When you criticize, do you tend to get sarcastic? Do you ever ridicule or laugh at your child's mistakes? How do you react when he makes a mistake? When you make a mistake? Do you put yourself down for your own shortcomings? Or do you see these—in yourself and in your child—as opportunities to grow, as challenges to be met? Do you see mistakes as disasters or as indicators of poor character, or do you see them as potential learning experiences? How you regard mistakes in yourself and in your child can have a big impact on your child's self-esteem.

Also, can you admit it when you make a mistake, especially when you're wrong and your child is right? Or do you need to seem perfect, need to be right, need to win all the time? If you take the risk of being human and imperfect with your teenager, it goes a long way in building self-esteem, helping to ease the teen's worries about his own imperfections and bridging any of the communication gaps you have between you.

Exercise: Think of the last time you made a mistake. How did you react? How did you resolve or rectify the matter? Next, consider your reaction when your teenager makes a mistake or falls short of a goal. What is your reaction then? Are you as hard or as gentle as you are with yourself? Did you label, criticize and scold or did you encourage him or her to meet the challenge of growing from the experience? How could you make it better the next time?

HOW DO YOU PRAISE YOUR TEENAGER? AND WHEN WAS THE LAST TIME YOU PRAISED YOUR TEEN?

Do you go for days, weeks or months without offering your teenager some encouragement? When you praise, what is his or her reaction? If the reaction is negative, take a look at the way you praise. Are you being honest in your praise?

Some teenagers quickly pick up on phony or manipulative compliments and are quick to discount any praise that doesn't ring true. It is counterproductive to praise your youngster only when you want him to do something for you, or to be unrealistic in what you say. If, for example, you tell your teenager who is doing well in art class that he is the greatest artist you've ever seen, you both know that this probably isn't true and the teen will feel patronized and put down. It is more productive to focus on progress—for example, "I really like that new watercolor you just finished. You seem to be enjoying the class and I'm so happy for you."

It's important to express praise the same way you express criticism—focusing on a specific quality of behavior, not the entire person. Focusing on the person and making a value judgment about his or her worth may lead the teen to believe that his goodness or personal worth is contingent on achievements or that your love is conditional on these.

For example, it is better to say, "I appreciate the way that you cleaned up the kitchen and washed the dishes tonight. That really helped a lot," instead of, "I love you for cleaning the kitchen. You're a great kid."

Or, when a teen has done something that took personal courage, it is more constructive to say quietly, "I'm so pleased you were able to get up in front of everyone and give such a good speech. I know you were nervous about it. You showed real courage," instead of, "I was bursting with pride! You're always so brave!"

The teen, who knows that he isn't always brave or thoughtful, will be pleased that you've noticed the progress and growth, but at the same time will realize that your love does not hinge on peak performances.

If you think that what you say doesn't matter, think again. No matter how tied teenagers are to their peers and how seemingly uninterested they are in you, your opinion matters a lot.

Exercise: Make an effort to give praise and positive feedback to your teenager in some way every day. It may be praise over some small matter ("I appreciate the way you started getting dinner ready on your own" or "It meant a lot to me when you asked me how things were at work today. It made me feel good to know that you're interested"). It takes time to listen to your teen—whether he or she is trying to tell you about a problem, a new friend at school, a hot news item or a very old joke. Making an effort to listen is a form of praise, since it is a way of saying to your child, "You're important to me."

Letting your child take more responsibility is also a form of praise because it implies trust and faith in his or her ability to take more control over life.

"Giving your teenager responsibilities, acting as if the teen can handle more, can help his self-esteem grow and give the teenager a sense of security, a wonderful feeling of being valued and trusted," says Dr. Doris Lion.

It isn't always easy to trust or to praise at first. If this isn't done openly in your family, you may feel a bit awkward and self-conscious at first. So often it's easier to hear and say negative things instead of positive things. Sometimes there may even be tears—surprised, relieved or joyful tears—when you praise. However difficult it may be at first, praising your teen is an excellent way to improve communication.

WHEN WAS THE LAST TIME YOU TOLD YOUR TEENAGER THAT YOU LOVED HIM OR HER?

Have you ever been able to do this? Some families are quite reticent about such feelings, and even spouses go for months or years without actually saying "I love you" to each other. But in families in which communication tends to be open, the various family members are able to say and to hear that they are loved and valued. When you're locked into conflicts with your teenager or when he or she is acting in a distinctly unlovable way, it is very difficult to summon up these feelings and words. But such times are when your teenager may need those words the most. There are times when your expressed love and commitment are what keep communication going between you.

Exercise: Tell your teenager that you love him or her sometime today. Or, if that is too difficult right now, you might write a note and leave it in his room telling the teen how much you love him—in good and bad times and for himself, not for what he does or doesn't do. If a teenager knows this, he or she will feel a renewed sense of self-worth and, perhaps, a new bond with you as well. If your teenager knows that your love is unconditional, trust, respect and better communication are more likely to grow.

DOES YOUR TEENAGER FEEL THAT HE OR SHE BELONGS IN THE FAMILY?

A sense of belonging is important to self-esteem. Even though your teen chooses to spend a lot of time away from home and seems uninterested in family activities, make an effort to include him or her whenever feasible, giving the teen the option of participating or not.

It is also helpful to communication and your teenager's sense of self-worth to include him or her in your feelings. If you try to hide your pain and sadness, you're communicating several things: that you don't trust the teen's growing ability to cope, that you see him or her as a child in need of protection and that feelings of pain and sadness are somehow wrong and should be hidden. Including your adolescent in some of your feelings helps your teen feel close to you-the-person versus you-the-parent and also helps him or her to feel more comfortable and able to cope with his own pain.

"In being open, you make the teen an ally, not an enemy," says Dr. Richard MacKenzie. "It's important to admit it to your child when times are tough and when you're feeling sad."

Giving your teenager a voice in family decisions or asking for his opinion, even in small matters, will help give him or her the sense of belonging and importance so necessary for self-esteem.

"You might do this on an informal basis or utilize one mealtime a week to raise issues about what's happening in your lives," Dr. MacKenzie suggests.

It is also helpful to express your need to stay in touch with your teenager.

"You might say something like 'I see you growing up and living more and more outside our home,'" says Dr. MacKenzie. "'I really enjoy seeing you grow up and experience the world, but I miss you. I would like to spend some time with you. Let's do something together—go for a hamburger, go sailing, something like that.' Make it clear that this is *your* need."

Exercise: Make an effort to include your teenager in some special way today. Ask his opinion about something important to you or to the family and listen carefully to his reply without rejecting or discrediting it. Ask his opinion on a small matter or two that are of immediate concern (for example, what dessert to fix for the big family dinner coming up next weekend). Ask him or her to participate in a family activity or something with just the two of you. Or share a special thought or feeling—maybe your need to stay in touch.

Remember that a teenager with high self-esteem will be more willing to communicate and compromise and less vulnerable to destructive peer pressure as well as to severe bouts of depression. Helping your child build a positive self-image is an excellent preventive measure. And even if your communication has broken down, even if your home is one of ongoing crises and confrontations, even if your teenager is already depressed, your attempts to empathize and to change the environment to one that encourages communication will help you and your teenager reach out and start to get back in touch with each other.

10

The Most Important Step: Learn Good Communication Skills

Effective communication is an art, and there are some essential skills you should develop in order to get past communication barriers and start getting through to each other. This chapter describes these skills in detail.

Listening

Too often what passes for conversation is really a long-winded monologue or two simultaneous monologues with neither speaker being heard by the other. This can be particularly true of "conversations" between parents and teenagers—with arguments, interruptions, excuses, lectures and accusations all short-circuiting any real communication.

Listening is the first step away from this frustrating no-win cycle. If you learn to listen, you will learn a great deal about your teenager and probably about yourself as well. Your listening will also make your teenager aware of how much you care and will facilitate communication.

Many parents have a difficult time listening to their kids. One father's re-action to a counselor's comments about the importance of listening: "Why should I have to listen to all that garbage? I don't agree with any of it and I feel that my kid is screwing up his life. I want to talk some sense into his head before it's too late!"

If you really want to get through to your teenager, listening is the best first step. It does *not* mean agreeing. "It doesn't mean that you're giving in to your kids," says Dr. Gabrielle Carlson. "What it means is that you're giving credence to their right to express themselves openly. It can be hard to hear what they're saying, but it's important to make an effort to listen."

Listening without interrupting can be difficult but crucial. "No matter how strongly you dislike or disagree with what's being said, it's important to listen anyway," says Dr. Judith Davenport. "Keep back the 'but's,' the excuses, the attacks and the judgments. If you're serious about expressing the sentiment 'I love you no matter what' to your teenager, listening in this way is a good chance to prove it."

It's also vital not only to hear what's being said, but also to understand the message and let your teen know that you understand. This is called "active listening."

The value of active listening is that it clarifies the speaker's feelings and cuts down on misunderstandings and misinterpretations. Since teenagers are not always able to articulate exactly how they feel, active listening on your part will help them identify and express their thoughts and feelings more clearly. And you will find yourself becoming better able to understand the feelings behind their words.

The techniques of active listening may seem awkward at first, as you feed back to your teenager your understanding of what he or she says. This does not mean parroting back the teen's words, however; that can short-circuit communication in record time. The following dialogue is an example of unsuccessful communication due to faulty (parroting) active listening:

TEEN: I'm never going back to that school again! I can't stand it anymore! I'm so mad at my English teacher I could scream!

PARENT: You're never going back to that school because you can't stand it anymore. You're so mad at your English teacher that you could scream.

TEEN: That's what I *said*! Stop repeating every word I say. What are you trying to do anyway?

A more successful attempt at active listening might go something like this:

TEEN: I'm never going back to that school again! I can't stand it any-more! I'm so mad at my English teacher I could scream!

PARENT: Wow! You really sound angry and frustrated.

TEEN: Yeah, I am! You know what she did? She marked me way down on that essay I worked on so hard and felt so good about be-cause she thought my handwriting was messy. She said the essay itself was excellent, but she gave me a C minus anyway because of my handwriting. I tried to be neat. I just have bad handwriting, that's all.

PARENT: You feel she was very unfair in doing this.

TEEN: Yeah, I do. It isn't fair! There's got to be a way I can talk with her about this so she'll listen and start to give me a chance. I'm working so hard in that class.

PARENT: You think that there might be a way to let her see things from your point of view.

TEEN: For some reason she likes to have essays handwritten. But maybe I could ask if I could word-process mine. That would make it easier for both of us. What do you think, Dad? Worth a shot, huh?

PARENT: It sounds like you've come up with a reasonable solution. Let me know how it goes.

Contrast this with the way the conversation might have gone with a couple of communication blocks thrown in:

TEEN: I'm never going back to that school again! I can't stand it any-more! I'm so mad at my English teacher I could scream!

PARENT: Lower your voice! Stop overreacting! Now what happened *this* time?

TEEN: Oh, forget it!

PARENT: Come on, tell me.

TEEN: You know the essay I worked on so hard? The one that was *good*? Well, she marked it way down! I got a C minus on it and only—

PARENT: I'm sure she had good reasons for giving you that grade. She's the teacher and a much better judge of what's good than you are.

TEEN: But I don't think she was fair! She admitted that the essay itself was excellent but gave it a low mark because of my handwriting. I can't help it if my handwriting is bad. I tried to be neat. I don't think my whole essay should have been marked down because of my handwriting!

PARENT: Well, your handwriting is terrible. Your teacher is just trying to help you. How many times have I told you to work on it more? The problem with you is that you're just too stubborn and lazy to do anything about it. If you tried harder and learned to write better, you wouldn't have problems like this. It's as simple as that.

TEEN: (crying) I knew you wouldn't understand! I hate everybody!

In the last example, the conversation served no constructive purpose and simply reinforced the parent's and teen's negative views of each other. In the earlier, workable, active-listening example, the teen ventilated his anger, confided in his father and drew closer to him while working out his own possible solution to his problem.

Sometimes active listening means noticing your child's body language to pick up cues about feelings, then making an observation about this with a leading question and an offer of support.

For example, when Sandra Lowell discovered her thirteen-year-old daughter, Lisa, coming quietly home from school and slipping into the family room to sulk (quiet homecoming + sulk = trouble at school; sulking in the family room versus her own room = "Maybe I'd like to talk about it"), she could have reacted in a variety of ways.

If Sandra had used her old communication-blocking pattern of coming on strong with questions, she might have started a conversation that went like this:

SANDRA: What's the matter with you, Gloomy Gus? Something happen at school?

LISA: (sulking, no answer)

SANDRA: Did you have a bad day? Come on, tell me! What's the matter? Did Paula get on your case again? Didn't you get to see Rick after study hall? Did that math teacher give you trouble again. Talk to me!

LISA: I don't feel like it!

SANDRA: But I'm your mother. I care. Tell me what's wrong. It's good to get these feelings out into the open.

LISA: Not now.

SANDRA: Why not now? I have time. I'm here, ready and willing to listen. Is it so terrible you can't discuss it? Are you in trouble in any way? What could be so awful you can't tell me?

LISA: I didn't say it was something earth-shattering, I just said—

SANDRA: Is it because you think I wouldn't understand? I was a teenager once myself, you know.

LISA: Oh, *Mother,* please! Just leave me alone!

But on this particular occasion, Sandra didn't revert to her old ways. With an action plan involving active listening, Sandra chose to gently let Lisa know that her depressed mood was noticed and that she was there to listen if Lisa wanted to talk about her feelings:

SANDRA: Oh hi, honey. You slipped in so quietly I didn't even hear you.

LISA: (sulking, no response)

SANDRA: It looks like you had a rough day.

LISA: (sighs deeply, looks away)

SANDRA: Feel like talking about it?

LISA: (no answer, still sulking)

SANDRA: I get the feeling that something is the matter, but you don't feel like talking about it right now.

LISA: (looking away, nods slowly)

SANDRA: I understand, Lisa. But if you change your mind and want to talk with me, I'll be glad to listen. (With a warm touch on Lisa's shoulder, Sandra turns to go.)

LISA: (starts crying) Mommy . . . wait. I'm just feeling so down because . . .

If you're in a situation in which you're listening to your teen complain about you or your rules, nonjudgmental active listening helps clarify feelings and keeps the confrontation from getting out of hand and becoming nonconstructive.

"Listen and make it clear that you're hearing the teen's message," says Dr. Judith Davenport. "If you need more information, ask for it. Put some responsibility for the relationship onto the teenager. You might, for example, reply to a teenager's charge that you're an unreasonable perfectionist who expects too much of him with 'I hear you saying that I expect too much of you. I need more information about what makes you feel that way.' Then it's important to hear him out. If the teen says, 'You want me to go to Stanford, which I probably can't get into anyway. You want it because your friends will be impressed. What I want doesn't even count.' Look and see if there is any truth in that. If you find a grain of truth, you can decide how you want to change or manage your own behavior."

Sometimes brief, nonjudgmental comments (for example, "I see") give your teen a sense of being heard and understood. When you listen in this way, your teenager will be more inclined to grant you the same courtesy.

"I was leery of it at first," says Susan Shelley, the divorced mother of two teenage daughters. "But it worked. The first time I tried it, my older daughter raged in the door and started yelling about something. My response was 'You really sound angry and upset.' Kerry paused, mid-scream, and said, in a normal tone of voice, 'Yeah, I really am,' and proceeded to tell me why in a calmer, more reasonable way than usual. It was great. I'm not always good at active listening, and it doesn't always work so smoothly because we're all only human after all, but Kerry, Randi and I are able to communicate better now. They've started doing the same type of listening with me, entirely on their own. It pleases me to hear it."

As Susan explains, active listening—a skill that can be developed on your own or in family counseling—is not a panacea for all communication ills. There will be times when your child refuses to talk with you. In such instances it helps to realize that sharing can't be forced. Ask the adolescent if he or she wants to talk, gently express your willingness to listen and then back off. If your teen knows you respect his or her feelings and privacy needs yet are willing to listen and help if you can, he or she is more likely to come around eventually.

"A little space and time for reflection helps a lot," says Shirley Lackey. "I've found that most people in families would really like to talk with each other; they're just scared to take the first step."

Through active listening to each other, you and your teenager may be able to get past that first step. This is of particular importance to the family of a depressed teenager, who presents an especially tough communication challenge. "But a parent who can listen and validate the child's anger instead of immediately counterattacking will be able to help alleviate the child's depression," says Dr. Richard Brown.

Recognizing the reality and validity of a teen's feelings through active listening helps trust, communication and the teen's self-esteem grow even when he or she is depressed. Dr. Richard MacKenzie suggests, "Instead of the old line 'What do *you* have to be depressed about?' you might choose to respond in a more positive way. You might say, for instance, 'I admire the fact that you can admit that you're depressed. A lot of us try to run away from depression.' And then go on to help the teenager sort out his feelings and alternatives."

Give Clear Messages

It is important to express your feelings and needs directly rather than in a manner that might be interpreted as a personal attack, triggering an immediate defense reaction (a great communication blocker) from your teenager.

Say exactly what you mean in a constructive way, taking time to sort out and understand your feelings. You might discuss these first with your spouse, a friend or a counselor. "See what's going on in your own life," suggests Dr. Doris Lion. "Maybe you're seeing your child's problem as larger than it is because you are trying to work out your own problems through the child. Or maybe not. But it's a good idea to think about your part of the family problem and to realize what is yours and what is separate so you can express your feelings clearly to your child."

Giving clear messages means saying "I feel hurt when you are not honest with me" instead of "You're a liar"; or "I feel worried and sad when I see you drinking and skipping school. I fear for your safety and your future" instead of "You're a loser! Don't expect me to put up with this and support you for the rest of your life"; or "I feel worried when you're late coming home. I get very upset when you're two hours late and I don't hear from you because I sit here worrying about what might have happened to you" instead of "Late again! Do you know what time it is? You're so selfish and inconsiderate! Why didn't you at least call and say you'd be late?"

What the "I" message does is to state clearly the *parent's* problem with the adolescent's behavior (letting him or her know that such behavior has an impact on the parent) while focusing on the behavior without attacking the person.

The basic form of the "I" message ("I feel _____ when _____.") works well in a variety of situations. This does not mean, of course, that you will always be heard, that your teenagers will not attack you as a person or refuse to listen. But consistent use of clearly worded "I" messages helps improve communication by making your teenager feel less threatened and thus more amenable to reasonable discussions on important family issues.

It's important to give positive "I" messages as well, telling your teenager what behavior you enjoy and appreciate. For example, you might say, "I feel good when you stop to talk with me after you get home from school," or "I appreciated it when you were so patient with Grandma today. I know it's hard to listen to her sometimes and I'm so pleased to see you treat her with such thoughtfulness and gentleness," or "I feel so happy when I come home from work and find that you've started dinner already. That helps a lot. Thank you!"

By focusing on both positive and negative behavior, you give your teen a clear and nonthreatening view of which behaviors you feel are okay and which ones you consider to be problems. It is an excellent way to set limits and communicate a clear sense that you and your teen are separate people who nevertheless have great impact on each other's lives and so must learn to communicate and cooperate with each other.

Respect Each Other's Separateness

Giving clear "I" messages and determining ownership of specific problems is only the beginning. Recognizing and respecting each other's separateness is even more important. This means sharing opinions, not dictums from on high. It means not lecturing or assuming that your children will naturally share all of your values. While we always hope that our children will share the values most important to us, there is no law that says they must. And even though you may seem incredibly at odds now, remember that questioning your values and acting or speaking in opposition to them is part of the separation behavior of adolescence. Chances are that when your teenager grows up, he or she will share more values in common with you than he or she seems to do now. Or perhaps not, but that still doesn't mean that you can't love and respect each other.

You may find that your concept of what is best for your child will never match his or hers and that after making your own feelings and values clear, you must accept what can't be changed, giving your son or daughter the space to make many choices, decisions and mistakes.

"It is important to nurture your child and allow him to develop in the best way he can, allowing him to feel good about what he can do," says Dr. Gabrielle Carlson. "It's critical to determine what you really want for your child. Do you want him to be the best he can be? Or the best way *you* want? There is a big difference between the two, and some difficulty is in store for you if you feel that when your child disagrees with you he is rejecting you. You must both allow each other some freedom of choice."

"Your teenager may value qualities in himself that elude you, and it's important to respect them," says Dr. Doris Lion. "And, in turn, you may value things that matter little to the child."

Tolerance for differing points of view cuts down a great deal on the nit-picking that erodes communication. By concentrating on crucial issues and accepting the less important differences as evidence of your child's separateness, you keep the lines of communication open, you have a better chance of getting through to your teenager when it matters and you help foster feelings of mutual respect in your home. The fact is, your children aren't likely to respect you and your feelings and values if you show no signs of respecting and accepting theirs.

Set Limits and Resolve Conflicts Together

Tolerating different points of view and giving your teenager the space to be his or her own person does not mean that you should not set limits. Teenagers need freedom, but they also need the security of knowing what is expected of them and what absolute limits exist in their homes.

"There are certain things you don't have to and shouldn't accept," says Dr. Lion. "In fact, you need to set limits. In doing so, you are saying, 'I care about you. I can't control your behavior nonstop, but these are the things I *expect.*' Then invite your teen to share his negative or positive feelings about this. It's important to listen and be firm and consistent about what you expect from your son or daughter. Adolescents *want* limits. It's scary not to have them. In fact, some acting-out behavior is a way of searching and asking for limits."

While your teenager complains and argues about your limits, he or she may also feel that you care enough to stand firm, nose-to-nose with him, and that you will not give up or give in and say, "Oh, do what you want. I don't care."

Special-education teacher Mary Ann Dan has found limit setting to be a way of gaining new respect and closeness with her particularly difficult teenage pupils. "The whole reason I'm successful with these kids is that I care and I won't give up on them," she says. "They have been shuffled around with threats like 'If you don't behave, you'll have to go to . . . ,' but my class is the end of the line. When a student gets defiant and says, 'So throw me out!' my reply is 'No way are you getting out of here. You're going to stay here and things are going to change. You and I may end up wrestling each other to the mat. That's okay. I'll roll around on the floor with you if I have to.' When they get the picture and realize I mean it, they say, 'Oh . . . well . . . okay.' This approach, which parents can utilize in especially tough situations, has worked even with my most difficult students."

The limits you set should be clear and reasonable. Let the small stuff go. Concentrate on major conflicts and concerns.

Reasonable limits are ones you can live with, ones you will stick to consistently and ones that will help your teenager realize the necessity of cooperation and compromise as a member of a family and of society at large. However, if your limits fluctuate constantly or are unreasonable, they are no help to you *or* to your teenager.

Dr. Gabrielle Carlson recalls the story of one particular family she is seeing in therapy whose limit setting leaves something to be desired. "This couple alternately infanticizes and jumps on their teenage daughter," she says. "A major conflict recently has been her irresponsible use of the family car and the fact that she never gets home on time. To 'solve' this, her parents recently bought her a brand-new car! This is *not* a good or reasonable way to set a limit. This couple is having a hard time seeing that they are rewarding bad behavior."

The key to effective communication about limits and conflict resolution is cooperation. If your family gets into the habit of working out conflicts together, it will do wonders for communication and harmony.

"Too many family conflicts are seen in terms of winning and losing rather than communicating and resolving problems," says Dr. Lion. "But the family is a system. What affects one affects all. If things are going to get any better around your home, you need family cooperation in resolving conflicts."

How can you begin to get this cooperation?

First, dispense with the old win-lose method of resolving differences. For example, maybe your teenage daughter screams loud enough and stomps around the house long enough to wear down your resolve, and thus "wins" her point. And you lose, feeling angry at her and at yourself for not standing your ground. Or perhaps you see a problem and think up a solution you feel is best. Without listening to alternative ideas or plans for meeting with the same goals that your teenager might have, you insist that he or she accept and follow your plan to the letter. You win the confrontation, but lose in the long run as your teen's resentment and rebellion against your solution build.

In place of the win-lose method of resolving family problems, try a "no-lose" way of working things out. This method of family cooperation is taught in a number of parenting classes.

The "no-lose" method of conflict resolution works this way:

1. Identify the problems between you. It's helpful to make a list of behaviors you expect from your teen or that you can't live with. Invite your teenager to do the same with you.

For example, you expect your teenager to go to school, to keep his or her room reasonably clean, to do specific household chores, to speak to you in a civil tone of voice, to observe curfew rules and not to host parties at your home in your absence. Your teenager's expectations might be that you quit nagging about exactly when chores are done, respect his or her privacy (for example, not opening mail or reading diaries), speak in a civil tone of voice, not embarrass him or her in front of friends and get off his or her back about hair or style of dress.

Once these conflicts, wants and expectations are out in the open, you can sort through your alternatives.

2. Brainstorm with your teenager to find solutions to major conflicts. Write down all suggestions without commenting one way or the other about them. When all suggestions have been made, go through the list together, each saying which alternatives might be acceptable. This way, it is usually possible to hit on at least one or two compromises to each problem that everyone can live with.

For example, you might both agree to speak civilly to each other. You might agree to relax your standards of cleanliness for your teen's room as long as dishes and food are not left in there to fester and the door is kept shut so you don't have to look at it. Your teenager may agree to do all expected household chores within an agreed-upon time frame if you don't nag about it. You may agree to keep from constantly criticizing your teen's friends if your teenager will stop inviting them over when you're not home or so often that the family routine is upset.

This way, both parent and teen win a bit and compromise a bit. This exercise will help your teenager learn constructive ways of working out conflicts. He or she will also be more strongly motivated to follow through on the solutions and expectations because of having had a voice in making them.

3. Explore ways to implement your compromises and decisions. It's important to agree on how these rules and decisions will be enforced. In matters in which solutions are readily agreed upon and quite easy to implement, verbal agreements (and gentle "I"- message reminders if someone slips up later on) are usually enough. In particularly serious or recurring conflicts, some families find a written contract useful.

Carol Calladine, social worker, mother of four and author (with her husband, Andrew) of *Raising Siblings,* says that contracts have worked well in her own family during continuing conflicts centering on the use of the stereo, family car or television or the assignment of chores. The Calladine family has developed a special contract for use of the stereo. Drawn up and signed by each member of the family, this contract allows one-hour-a-day use of the stereo for each family member with a weekly sign-up sheet to ensure each person a specific daily time slot. Those who violate the terms of the contract lose use of the stereo for a week.

"Contracting is the big discipline gun in our family," Carol Calladine says. "We don't dilute it with overuse, but save it for repetitive problems or cooperation issues."

4. Give the agreed-upon compromises a fair trial. Follow your agreements for a week or two, then get together to discuss how they are working. If a solution is *not* working, you and your teen should reevaluate it and explore other possibilities. If it is working well, share your good feelings about that fact—and each other—and agree to continue.

Working out problems this way is not easy. Your teen may resist your efforts and refuse to compromise, reverting to old behavior patterns such as tantrums, sulking or retreating. In such instances it helps to hang in there. Give your teenager a clear, firm message that these tactics will no longer work with you, that you feel angry at such behavior and that you expect him or her to meet you halfway. Given the choice between compromise or continuing conflict, a teenager will often come around.

5. Make time for each other. Working out conflicts, giving each other clear messages and getting to know each other as unique individuals take time. Give high priority to making time to communicate with your teenager not only about conflicts and expectations, but also about happy, positive feelings and observations. Choose communication time wisely. Trying to snag your teenager for a talk when he or she is dashing out the door is counterproductive. You both need time to express feelings—to listen, share and really connect with each other—without one eye on the clock or the TV screen or one foot out the door. If your lives are very busy and heavily scheduled, make a date with one another, giving yourselves time without distractions or pressure to communicate.

Making time for each other on a regular basis gives you a chance to share all kinds of feelings and myriad experiences. Sharing vulnerabilities—laughing together, crying together, enjoying good times and hanging in through the rough times—does a lot to strengthen your relationship. Seeing each other as people rather than as constant adversaries aids your communication tremendously, but this takes time and many shared feelings to accomplish.

Making time to have fun together and to enjoy each other between all the pain and conflict that adolescence may bring to your family keeps your bonds strong and the lines of communication open even in the midst of a serious crisis. The memories of your good times together and your love for each other will sustain you and your teen through a lot of storms.

6. Seek help if you can't get through to each other. Cultivating good communication is often a considerable challenge and may be impossible to do without professional help, especially if your family is in a serious crisis or your teenager is extremely depressed.

"I always stress the importance of a parent establishing an open line of communication with a depressed teenager, but I do this with some hesitation," says Dr. Richard MacKenzie. "The problem is that depressed kids usually don't like to talk much and it may be that they will find it easier to talk with a non-parental adult: a nurse, teacher, physician, minister or counselor. You may need to look for outside help in order to get through to each other."

Professional help (from a psychiatrist, psychologist, social worker, family or youth counselor or clergyperson) may be necessary, especially if your teen is severely depressed or acting out in destructive ways—with alcohol or drug abuse, for example.

"Unfortunately, there are no set rules for helping a teenager through a crisis, no seven-rule strategy for constructive coping," says Dr. Alan Berman, "It may be helpful to get therapy, to get both your teenager and yourself involved, making it clear that you're doing this because you care. It's important to realize that instant results are unlikely. It took some time for the current problems to develop, and it's likely to take some time to sort things out. A professional therapist will help you to explore the dynamics of your problems with each other, how these came to be and how you might begin to help and change the situation."

Whether or not you need outside help in breaking down the communication barriers you and your teenager have built up over the years, getting back in touch with each other takes time. It will be a struggle. But effective, loving communication helps to *prevent* depression from becoming a major problem for your teenager and your family. Most of all, breaking down communication barriers can help you get to know, have compassion for and enjoy each other better and more often. Growing in communication skills will give all of you a lifetime of rewards.

Part IV

WHAT TO DO WHEN YOUR TEEN IS HAVING SCHOOL PROBLEMS

11

Your Teen and School Problems

School looms large as both a cause and a stage for symptoms of teenage depression and anxiety.

Perhaps your teen suddenly won't go to school, claiming that he or she is afraid of violence or of ridicule.

Perhaps your teen, previously an excellent student, seems to have lost all interest and motivation—and his or her grades are starting to show a downward spiral.

Perhaps your teen is experiencing sudden difficulties: not getting along with longtime friends or feeling unable to make friends at all and hopeless about anything changing.

Perhaps your teen has a learning disability that is at the heart of his lack of confidence and is feeling increasingly different from peers and uncomfortable at school.

It could be, too, that you're not sure what is going on—only that your teen's school experience is changing in troubling ways.

Sometimes this is due to a change of schools, particularly the transition from elementary school to junior high. In this transition, many young adolescents can lose confidence, motivation and interest. Studies have found that the environment of junior high—with greater teacher control, fewer positive student-teacher relationships, higher performance expectations and escalating peer pressure—often comes at the same time (especially for girls) that the physical and emotional changes of puberty are at their height.

On the other hand, recent studies have found that young adolescents who are enrolled in schools with K–8 configurations and are not faced with a change of schools until the age of fourteen or so are much less likely to suffer from falling grades, interest and motivation. This could be because they are well into puberty—and through the most unsettling part of adolescent changes—before they have to make an additional adjustment to a new school setting.

Schools are also changing. They feel less safe to teens today for a variety of reasons: escalating violence, assaults and on-campus killings, and increased awareness of sexual harassment. In an informal 1993 *USA Today* poll of 65,193 young people in grades six through twelve, more than one-third reported feeling unsafe at school, up from almost one-quarter in 1989. Half of those polled knew someone who carried a weapon to school and half also knew someone who had switched schools to feel safer. Some 43 percent reported avoiding restrooms because of fear for their safety, and 63 percent felt that they would learn more if they felt safe at school.

Concurrent with these changes in teens' school experiences is the unchanging fact of pressure to succeed. Adult pressures—to make good grades, to get into a good college—continue. And, as always, bright teens put pressure on themselves to do well.

School problems can be a catalyst for teenage depression. If a teen feels rejected by peers or labeled and limited by a learning disability, or if a teen is stressed out or harassed or unsafe at school, he or she is susceptible to depression.

On the other hand, signs and symptoms of depression may be most evident as a teen withdraws from peers, loses motivation, gets into conflicts with classmates or teachers or refuses to go to school altogether.

Why is school so often both a source and a stage for symptoms of depression?

School is one area over which the teen has a certain amount of control. While you may control finances, family lifestyle and domicile, curfews and the like, a teenager has a wide range of choices regarding his or her academic career. He often chooses whether or not to achieve to the best of his ability, to work hard, to get into trouble at school. Because of this, teenagers often use school achievement or nonachievement to assert their independence and to test limits.

School is also a handy and noticeable stage for acting out. While sulking around the house may be ignored, denied or relegated to the category of normal teenage behavior by the parent, a notice from school about behavioral, academic or attendance problems is usually a surefire parental attention getter. It's a way of telling adults there's definitely something the matter even if the teenager himself isn't quite sure what the trouble might be.

Finally, school is a considerable source of stress for kids and as such may be the breaking point for a depressed teenager. Attending a huge junior high or high school may be an alienating experience. And as performance expectations escalate, so do stress, anxiety and depression. School is more important to many teens than adults imagine. In his study of adolescent priorities, Dr. Aaron Hess, a psychologist at UCLA School of Medicine, surveyed 625 high school students and discovered that doing well in school was the number one priority for boys and the number two priority for girls. If a teenager has a learning disability, low self-esteem or emotional or family problems that make it more difficult to meet academic challenges, a self-perpetuating cycle of depression and school problems can result.

What kinds of school-related problems are depressed teenagers likely to have? Most fall into six general categories:

Lack of motivation: This is manifested by a loss of interest and momentum in school, falling grades, loss of involvement in extra-curricular activities or problems with teachers and peers.

Learning disabilities: These include not only common ones such as dyslexia and attention-deficit disorder, but also learning problems that may stem from the side effects of medications or chronic diseases. Whatever the source, having a learning disability can put a teen at risk for depression at a time when it's distressing to be different from peers.

Serious problems with teachers, peers and/or school authorities: Some troubled teenagers get into angry confrontations and fights with teachers, school officials or classmates. Or they get into trouble because of other behavior such as drug or alcohol abuse. Or they may be so withdrawn and unable to relate to those around them that this becomes a problem in itself and may certainly be a symptom of depression. It is the quiet, withdrawn teenager no one notices who is most likely to commit suicide. So *not* relating to others can be as serious a symptom as fighting.

Achievement stress: This can hit the best and the brightest adolescents with sometimes devastating results. Feeling pushed by teachers, parents and themselves, some talented, achieving teens feel that their entire self-worth, and perhaps parental love, is based on their continuing achievement—and that is why a stumble along the path, a setback or a failure can feel like a disaster and in some instances have health or life-threatening consequences.

School phobia: This is a tendency to avoid school via myriad symptoms, crises and excuses, including a constant array of physical complaints; expressed fears of peers, teachers or the school setting; crying; temper tantrums; oversleeping; withdrawal and stubborn refusal to attend classes on a regular basis. "Teens who have concurrent depression and anxiety are particularly likely to exhibit school phobia and school avoidance."

Truancy: Unlike the phobic teen, the habitual truant isn't necessarily afraid of school or distraught at the idea of attending. He or she just isn't interested in what school has to offer and can think of many more appealing things to do than going to classes.

Do any of these situations have a ring of familiarity? The rest of this chapter will look at these common problems in detail and offer some suggestions about how you, as a parent, can help to alleviate your teen's depression-based school problems or his or her school-exacerbated depression.

Lack of Motivation

Thirteen-year-old Jennifer Siegal was an excellent student in elementary school, but the picture is changing now that she is an eighth-grader at a large suburban junior high school. Her parents have noticed a major change in her attitude and in her grades this year. "She doesn't seem to care," says Myra Siegal. "She procrastinates, sleeps a lot and then frantically rushes to get assignments done at the last minute—if she does them at all. She used to be an A student. Now she's just getting by. We got a notice the other day that she's close to failing two classes. I've tried to find out what problems she's having, but she just says she doesn't know what's the matter. It's so frustrating because my husband and I *want* to help, but we don't know how, or what to do!"

Jennifer Siegal's dwindling interest in school and her falling grades are fairly typical of the lack of motivation that can strike adolescents, especially in junior high school. This loss of academic motivation is often due to depression—or to factors that can make a teen vulnerable to depression.

Some non-depressed teenagers also lose motivation at this time because they are overwhelmed by developmental and social changes occurring at the same time as the transition to junior high, which, as we have seen, can be a particularly difficult one. With their rapidly changing bodies and their growing interest in romantic/sexual feelings and experiences and in being an accepted member of their peer group, some teenagers—at least temporarily—don't have the energy or inclination to devote as much time to school and studies. Added to that, the transition to junior high can be unsettling and overwhelming.

"They go from a small and personal elementary school to a much larger school," says educational psychologist Sarah Napier. "Suddenly, everything is depersonalized. Teachers don't know them in quite the same way. Some kids feel like a number on a roll sheet and don't quite feel that they belong."

While most adolescents eventually adjust and are able to get back to a consistent level of academic performance after a temporary drop in grades and interest, there are some teens who continue to have problems.

For some teenage girls, loss of motivation may be linked to the mixed messages that young women get from teachers, friends and society in general. The messages they get in school can hit particularly hard. A 1993 study conducted by the Wellesley College Center for Research on Women found that girls are treated as second-class citizens in junior high and senior high classrooms—given less attention and affirmation than boys—and that textbooks too often ignore or stereotype women.

Girls who are more physically mature have a particularly difficult junior high school experience and are more vulnerable to a variety of problems, according to another 1993 study, conducted by Dr. Jacquelynne S. Eccles and her colleagues at the universities of Colorado and Michigan. This study found that early-maturing females reported less opportunity to participate in classroom decision making, that teachers do respond differently to students in the same classroom depending on a variety of characteristics and that it is also possible for students to perceive the same classroom environment in a variety of ways. The study found that more physically mature female adolescents had a much more difficult time fitting into the junior high environment and experienced more school problems and truancy than their male classmates or their less physically mature female classmates.

Many girls, whatever their level of physical maturity, may lose interest in achievement when they hit puberty, sensing that competing successfully with male classmates might be a detriment to popularity or be regarded as unfeminine. Despite all the advances that women have made in the past two decades, such perceptions linger and are reinforced by peers and by the popular media. Studies of popularity criteria have found again and again that competency and leadership qualities make a teenage boy popular, while prettiness, thinness and nice clothes are the top popularity factors for girls.

Some unmotivated teens may have negative role models. Perhaps their closest friends don't assign much importance to academic pursuits and achievements. Maybe parents don't or can't act as models for hard work and persistence. These would include not only parents who have chronic problems with work and motivation themselves, but also parents who, after a lifetime of hard work and achievement, find themselves victims of nineties-style corporate downsizing and the economic recession, and are unemployed or underemployed. Some teens wonder about the value of striving for academic achievement and professional success when such success and security can be so elusive.

Stressful life events can also have an impact on school performance in young adolescents. A 1992 study reported in *Contemporary Pediatrics* lists parental death, divorce, remarriage, the birth of a sibling and a household move as major factors in declining school performance. Quite often such declines occur along with stress and depression accompanying such life events.

Still other teens have difficulty linking current efforts with future goals—goals that seem so far away. Many classes, from algebra to history, seem to have little to do with skills a teen wants to develop or distant goals he wants to meet. And so for a time the adolescent may coast.

How can you tell if your teen's lack of motivation stems from depression or from environmental factors and whether it will be temporary or lingering and possibly life-changing?

The situational lack of motivation is less likely to be accompanied by other symptoms or problems in most cases and is not as drastic a departure from the youngster's previous behavior. For example, a former A student, unsettled by the transition to junior high or upset over a parental divorce or a family move, may slip a bit in grades and academic interest but will usually not fail a class or have persistent academic difficulties unless overwhelmed by depression or other emotional problems.

Learning Disabilities and Other Academic Problems

Christopher Frank, twelve, has been struggling with depression, loneliness and a sense of isolation that have combined to make his seventh-grade transition from elementary school to junior high a crisis. Diagnosed with attention-deficit disorder some years ago, he has been in special-education classes since second grade and never seemed to mind. Now he feels labeled by schoolmates for being in "the dummy classes" and, in a desperate attempt to fit in, has been spending his allowance on treats that he distributes to peers, hoping to win their approval. His efforts have been met with contempt. His school counselor fears that he may be having some suicidal feelings and suggests that he transfer to another junior high in the district where he can get off to a fresh start with counseling guidance and parental support. But his mother, Glenda, has one nagging fear. "What if it isn't any different at the new school?" she asks, tears welling in her bright blue eyes. "What then?"

For a teenager with a learning disability or even one who simply struggles to keep up academically with classmates or with higher-achieving siblings, there can be a cyclical relationship between inability to keep up academically and low self-esteem and depression.

Some teens feel isolated and labeled by their special needs. Others feel hopeless facing a constant stream of daily struggles and disappointments and wondering if anyone knows how hard they are trying. Still others, who may or may not have learning disabilities, feel that they can never measure up to siblings or friends held up as examples of achievement by teachers or by parents.

School can be a daily ordeal for a learning-disabled teen and he may be less able and less likely to console himself with dreams that things will be better in the future, making it more difficult to pass up quick fixes and short-term pleasures for long-term goals.

Other teens struggle with learning problems that may be linked with chronic illnesses that can also have a negative impact on an adolescent's self-esteem. For example, recent research has found that in general, diabetic children and teenagers are twice as likely as nondiabetic classmates to have learning problems, and that diabetic boys are most likely of all to struggle, with 40 percent of the boys studied requiring special attention from teachers or needing to repeat a grade.

For a variety of reasons, which we will explore in later chapters, teens with diabetes and epilepsy are at particular risk of depression because their special medical needs make them feel different from peers.

It's important to keep in mind with students who struggle that a learning disability does not necessarily mean low intelligence and that there are many different kinds of intelligence. Some young people who may struggle with reading or writing or math might have strong abilities in other areas—from sports or dance to social savvy. These strengths need to be emphasized even as the learning problems are addressed.

Peer Rejection and Other Relationship Difficulties

As we saw in Chapter 2, peer rejection or harassment can be a factor in teenage depression and school problems. Sometimes a depressed teen may get into conflicts with peers, prompting rejection or ridicule. Other teens get depressed because they feel rejected by schoolmates. Many times it's hard to tell what began the cycle of misery—peer difficulties or depression.

Some teens can feel depressed and hopeless as the result of difficulties with a particular teacher or school official.

"My son Mike had a seventh-grade math teacher who just seemed to hate him on sight, and Mike developed an attitude in that class and it was just aw-ful for a while," Sharon Davis remembers. "There were some mornings when it was all I could do to get him to go to school. He got very depressed and felt pretty hopeless about changing anything. He was doing fine in his other classes and had good friends, but that one teacher's dislike really weighed heavily on him."

Some teachers—like peers—may have adverse reactions to kids who are smart but bored, who are shy and withdrawn or who have a problem that seems to be without a solution.

People tried to be nice to fourteen-year-old Jacquie Marshall when she started ninth grade, but it wasn't easy: The depressed, obese teenager sabotaged any attempt to help her develop an exercise and nutrition regimen that would help her physically; she refused emotional help and support from the school counselor, and she was mean to classmates who tried to befriend her. Soon people—her classmates and teachers—began to defend themselves and their own failure with Jacquie by making jokes about her behind her back. Needless to say, this only increased her depression and the hopelessness of her situation.

Achievement Stress

Marissa Chu's crying spells and moments of despair belie her outstanding school achievements: science awards, top grades, overtures from highly selective colleges. "Sometimes I feel I don't have a life," she says, twisting a crumpled tissue around in her hands. "I feel like my whole life depends on what I do in my senior year and that everything, including my parents' hopes for me, hinges on my getting into Harvard. I'm so scared of failing. It would feel like dying to me."

The teenager who feels that his entire future and even parental love hinge on his achievements, or who feels unable to live up to high family expectations, is at great risk for depression and potential school problems.

"I see students all the time from private prep schools and one public school for gifted students who feel that if they don't keep a perfect GPA and get into an Ivy League college, their lives will be over," says Dr. Charles Wibbelsman, who has given lectures on achievement stress for parents of students in these schools as one way of addressing the problem. "Sometimes the pressure makes these highly responsible kids go over the edge into depression, eating disorders and even suicidal behavior. I saw a teenager in the emergency room this past weekend who is a top student at a local prep school. He got so stressed out that he spent the weekend in Haight-Ashbury taking every pill you can imagine. By the time I saw him, he was unconscious and having seizures. We don't know yet what his ultimate prognosis will be. Even though this is an extreme example of a bright teen reacting adversely to stress, it's a red flag that this pressure can be life-threatening."

What many of these teens and their parents need to know is that there is more to life than grades—even the most selective colleges say so. Ivy League and other highly selective colleges do pay attention to grades, of course, but they also pay a tremendous amount of attention to extracurricular activities, charity activities, essays that show creative expression and personal integrity and recommendations that give a more well-rounded view of the individual. And, of course, bright teens need to know that life is not over if they don't get into the college of their choice.

"Mallory was distraught when she didn't get into Northwestern," says Frank Watson of his now nineteen-year-old daughter. "All through high school, her goal was to go to Northwestern's journalism school. But she didn't get in. She thought it was the end of the world. But we convinced her to enroll in the college that did offer her admission—the University of California, Santa Cruz. It's perfect for her. Now we know that the more intense academic atmosphere at Northwestern would have been all wrong for her."

Self-imposed pressure to fit an idealized image, the inability to reach this ideal and the tendency to link self-worth with achievement can cause an adolescent to burn out and sink into depression.

"Feeling that you *are* your work immobilizes you," says Dr. Barry Schwartz, a psychiatrist in Bala Cynwyd, Pennsylvania. "The student feels, for example, that when a paper is being graded, *he* is being judged and graded. This leads to procrastination and even complete immobilization. If a student's self-worth and self-image depend on what he does, he'll end up able to do nothing. Such a teenager must realize that what he produces is something he does, but it is not him and that there are many wonderful qualities he has that can't be measured academically."

How You Can Help

TALK WITH YOUR TEENAGER IN A NONJUDGMENTAL WAY

Using "I" statements, express your concern and ask for more information from your son or daughter:

"I notice that you seem to be having trouble in school lately and I'm concerned for you. How can I help?"

"I've been concerned because you seem lonely and upset at this new school. If you'd like to talk about it, I'm here for you."

"Sometimes I get the feeling that you feel you are your achievements and that you might feel Dad and I expect you to be number one in everything when we really just want you to be happy being yourself. Can we talk about this? I worry that you may be under too much stress about all this."

If your teenager is willing and able to share his or her feelings with you, you may get some valuable clues about what is happening and how best to help. With active listening, you may be able to help your teen explore constructive alternatives.

COMMUNICATE UNCONDITIONAL LOVE TO YOUR TEENAGER

Depressed teenagers feeling pressure by high parental expectations often feel that parental love and their own personal worth are contingent on fulfilling these expectations. Expressing your love for your child and making a verbal distinction between your love for her personally and your pride or concern over what she does can help your teenager to make the essential separation between who she is and what she does and to feel more valued and cherished as a whole person. Help your teenager realize that while achievements give some satisfaction, these don't serve to justify her existence. Help your teen understand that she would still be the same person and loved just as much without top grades, honors and prizes.

PRAISE THE EFFORT, NOT JUST THE RESULTS

Especially for teens with learning problems, it's vital that you give recognition and praise for their efforts. If your teen knows that you recognize and appreciate how hard he is trying and that a C for him may be as hard-won as an A for a sibling, he will be more likely to sustain hope and motivation.

Even with teens who are achievers, praising the effort is a way of letting them know that you realize how hard they are working—and that their success is very much their own.

LET YOUR TEEN "OWN" PEER PROBLEMS, BUT FIND A SOLUTION TOGETHER

If your teen is having relationship problems at school with peers or a teacher, don't take over the problem and rush to intervene with the parties involved. Listen carefully to what's going on with your teen and then ask him what he thinks might help. If he's feeling hopeless, explore some possibilities, giving him the freedom to accept whatever choices seem most reasonable to him. In some cases, role-playing a tough situation—to build his confidence in dealing with relationship problems or to model a more effective approach—can help. In other cases, helping him acquire essential social skills can go a long way toward helping your teen help himself.

HELP YOUR TEENAGER REDUCE STRESS

This means helping your son or daughter identify and value other areas of strength—personal qualities, interesting hobbies, creative talents and the like—that cannot be measured academically. Help your teenager to explore reasonable goals. Encourage her to get regular physical exercise and to pursue some hobbies and activities just for fun. Make sure that she has some amount of unstructured time and is not overscheduled. Relaxation, friends and hobbies can be important in reducing stress.

It is also helpful to communicate to your child the importance of seeing setbacks and mistakes in a new way. "The young person must learn that even when he fails at something, it is *not* the end of the world," says Dr. Bruce

Bongar, a clinical psychologist who has taught burnout-prevention classes to college students in the Los Angeles area. "We learn from our mistakes as well as our successes."

Encouraging your teenager to talk about fears, feelings and experiences and listening actively as he talks also helps to reduce his stress level and depression. When brought out into the open and discussed, many fears lose their impact, and seemingly impossible problems turn out to have a number of alternative solutions worth exploring. Just getting some feelings off his or her chest makes a difference for the teenager, and hearing these feelings gives you a chance to clarify any misunderstandings and misconceptions and modify your own behavior if need be.

HELP YOUR TEENAGER TAKE MORE CONTROL OVER HER LIFE

For a teen with a learning disability, this can mean providing the structure necessary for her to make the best use of her time and strengths. Let her know what you expect and when, and specifically what she needs to do step-by-step to accomplish these goals. Then offer praise and encouragement at each step.

In general, if you communicate to your teen that you really want what's best for her and that ultimately she is responsible for each choice, you will help defuse nonachievement as a potent weapon. Many teenagers, too, can't see long-range consequences of present actions. Melissa, for example, is a fourteen-year-old who talks about wanting to go to medical school but who is unwilling to go to classes now because she is bored, hates her science teacher and has no real friends.

With a teen such as Melissa, a helpful approach might be to suggest that together you explore ways to change these immediate concerns. This could mean finding interesting outside pursuits or doing extra-credit work if schoolwork isn't sufficiently challenging, learning to cope constructively with her science teacher (developing the knack for getting along with difficult people is an important life skill) or, if the teacher's truly impossible, switching classes or simply toughing it out.

If a teenager is discouraged because some classes seem meaningless, it helps to explore ways that such things relate to future goals and effectiveness—whether by giving one a broader understanding of human nature or by enabling one to develop necessary survival skills such as discipline, flexibility and patience. Helping your teen find the opportunities for growth that exist in unpromising classes may ease some of her disenchantment.

It is helpful, too, to show interest in your teenager's short- and long-range plans and goals and to encourage her to plan for the future.

Putting responsibility for life planning on your teenager while offering warm support and encouragement can help a great deal. If your teen has seemingly unrealistic goals—such as being a movie star or a rock idol—it is important to listen to these without disparaging them.

If your teen has very limited aspirations, a tactful lead-in to further discussion may be in order. It would be a good idea to find out her special strengths and abilities and develop certain skills to help her cope with whatever comes her way. If you keep your comments nonjudgmental and gently suggest that she take primary responsibility for setting goals, your teen will be more receptive to your ideas and your help in exploring possibilities.

Encouraging your teen to begin taking control of his life and to explore strengths, talents, prospects and possibilities helps a depressed teenager to realize that there *is* hope, that chances for change do exist and that he may actually have the power—and your loving support—to make some positive changes in his life. This is a crucial turning point in developing motivation to cope successfully with the challenges that come his way.

"All kids make a very serious internal decision about the time they are thirteen to sixteen years old," says special education teacher Mary Ann Dan. "It is a decision that they are or aren't going to be able to take care of themselves in life. The ones who decide that they *are* going to cope go to school, look forward to holding a job and learn the skills of establishing and maintaining good relationships with others. The ones I see in my classroom have decided that they are not going to care for themselves. They have fantasies of living off the land, in the woods or on welfare, usually via getting pregnant or getting a girl pregnant. Motivating teenagers to take care of themselves at this crucial age makes a great difference in their life—now and in the future."

CHAPTER

12

School Phobia

It began with an escalating array of physical complaints: stomachaches, headaches, cramps, fever or fatigue that precluded her getting up and getting ready for school on time. There have been times recently when fourteen-year-old Kerry McElroy cries, screams and simply refuses to go to school. Her bewildered parents report that it seems that she's terrified to go to school, but can't give any real reason for it.

"My wife, Nancy, and I both work, and this morning battle, added to our tight schedules, is truly wearing us down," says her father, Don McElroy. "If we leave before Kerry does in the morning, we *know* she won't go to school. She seems unable to cope with school and we're less and less able to cope with her inability to cope. Frankly, we're stumped at the moment."

While Kerry McElroy's sudden aversion to school is bewildering and frustrating to her parents, her behavior is not unusual. In fact, it is estimated that school phobia—an irrational, persistent fear of going to school—afflicts about one percent of all students at some point in their academic careers.

Why does school phobia happen?

These days there are many who would argue that school phobia is completely rational given the alarming increase in campus violence in the past few years. But there is a major difference between rational and irrational fears. A student who is quite reasonably afraid will be able to state his or her fears clearly. The teen suffering from school phobia may not be able to tell you why the prospect of going to school is so frightening.

School phobia can develop as the result of severe depression, which immobilizes the teenager and makes him feel that he can't possibly cope with the pressures and challenges of school. It can also develop as the result of an escalation of a number of fears and stressors. These combine to make school seem an impossible burden to a shy, sensitive, insecure adolescent.

Dr. Bettie B. Youngs, on the faculty of the department of educational administration at San Diego State University, conducted a study in which she examined common student stress factors that contribute to depression, shyness, phobias and hostility to authority. Among the stress factors she identified: fear of undressing in the gym locker room; fear of coming to terms with/exposure of one's sexuality (this would be especially true with teens who are gay or who are identified by peers as possibly gay); fear of being picked first (and having to lead) or last (which can be interpreted as being rejected or being unpopular) for a team or project; fear of confrontations with teachers; fear of getting poor grades (or of not making top grades); fear of participating in athletics and failing; fear of being ridiculed by peers, especially in the classroom when asked to speak; and fear of peers viewing one's physical self in a negative way—as fat, skinny or ugly.

A special problem with one stressor or with a combination of these can add up to a stubborn case of school phobia. Adolescent medicine specialist Dr. Charles Wibbelsman reports that he has seen teens who break into tears and say that they can't possibly go to school or participate in gym class, for example, because they're too embarrassed to undress in front of classmates. "In junior high especially there is such a wide range of normal physical development and a lot of noticeable differences," he says. "These differences are very significant to adolescents, and if one feels he or she is less developed than classmates, it is very threatening to undress in the locker room and expose this fact to everyone."

Some teens become disinclined to go to school in order to avoid a certain class. Kim Fisher, for example, began developing headaches and missing several days of school a week soon after beginning her sophomore year of high school. The major factor behind her school phobia seemed to be a difficult and demanding geometry teacher.

"It just got worse and worse," says her mother, Mary. "She was so afraid of this nun, who yelled at students if they gave wrong answers or asked questions. She didn't dare ask questions. Her fear got in the way of her understanding the class material and she wasn't doing well. She was so afraid of getting yelled at for making a mistake that she avoided going to school whenever possible, which meant that she got further and further behind."

Some teenagers avoid school out of fear of their peers. Linda Jamison, fourteen, whose stomachaches have kept her out of classes a large amount of time lately, complains that a group of girls keep chasing her and threatening to beat her up. Her parents observe that these disabling stomachaches never hit on weekends or school holidays.

And some young people are afraid to go to school because they feel responsible for holding things together at home. Sixteen-year-old Paul Smith confessed to a school counselor that he was afraid to go to school because his alcoholic father might physically harm his mother.

School phobia springs from a multitude of causes and too often parents unwittingly encourage it by making special demands or by allowing their teens to stay home day after day, thus reinforcing the phobia.

How You Can Help

Even though the situation seems to be at an impasse, with your teenager either actively or passively refusing to go to school because of fear, along with physical and emotional upsets, there are a number of things you can do to help.

EXAMINE THE REASONS BEHIND YOUR CHILD'S PHOBIA

Try to communicate your concern and encourage your teenager to talk about the feelings and the fears behind this sudden school phobia. Encourage your teen to be specific—not just offering comments such as "People tease me" or "Someone is going to get me." You need to know more about the circumstances, the people involved and how long this has been going on before you can begin to help.

Just getting some of the teen's fears and feelings out into the open is an important step in resolving the phobia.

LISTEN ACTIVELY

Give your teenager the feeling that what he says is important. Don't disparage, ridicule, contradict or criticize any of the fears or feelings your child expresses. They may seem irrational, but they're painful and real. Allowing your adolescent to talk freely will defuse some of this fear and help him problem-solve and discover possible solutions via this "thinking out loud" process.

HELP YOUR TEEN EXPLORE NEW ALTERNATIVES

Some possible alternatives might be a change in the teen's own behavior and attitudes at school or toward herself.

Carol Holmby, fourteen, was reluctant to go to school because she said that everyone picked on her and made fun of her because she was tall and slightly overweight, and some classmates even followed her around, teasing her until she cried. With her parents' gentle help, Carol explored ways that she could change the situation. "Since you can't directly change someone else's behavior, can you think of some things you can do to keep people off your back?" her mother asked.

"Not give them the satisfaction of seeing me upset?" Carol suggested. Then the family discussed the fact that perhaps refusal to accept the role of victim and failure to act in predictable ways would help Carol's situation. Her father suggested that she throw her tormentors off balance by agreeing with them: "Yes, you're right. I'm fat. And you wouldn't believe how clumsy I am!" Then he suggested that she might ignore them. The point was to act in an unpredictable way that would confuse her attackers, make them feel silly and not give them the satisfaction of visibly upsetting her.

Carol and her parents also discussed the fact that no one can be liked by everyone despite the unrealistic expectations and desires for universal popularity we all occasionally have. Together they made a list of important people in their lives, people they loved and valued and who returned these feelings. They also made lists of people they would like to get to know better. Carol listed three possible new friends at school and decided that cultivating these few important relationships would be very high on her priority list, while relegating the negative people to a less important role in her life.

Carol didn't solve all her problems through this discussion, but it was a great help in giving her the confidence to try to make changes in her way of acting and reacting at school.

Through active listening and gentle support, Richard Lawrence helped his son Mark work through his fears about undressing in the locker room. Mark, who is small and relatively undeveloped for a thirteen-year-old, seemed reassured when his father told him that he, too, had gone through these fears and feelings as a late bloomer, that late development is often genetically linked and that his stage of development was normal for him. Mark, who had been worried that he was *not* normal and would never grow and develop, was relieved to hear this and said that he felt better about his body. Having made this step, Richard and his son discussed ways that Mark might feel more comfortable about undressing for gym. Together they came to the conclusion that this was a threatening situation for most young teens and that maybe the people who were quick to ridicule were also feeling insecure and needed to build themselves up by tearing others down.

In exploring possibilities with your teenager, be sensitive to his or her reservations. If your teenager says, "Yes, but . . ." to a suggestion or observation, be supportive of this feeling with a response such as: "I get the feeling that you have reservations about that suggestion. That's fine. Let's talk about these reservations and some other ideas for changing the situation for the better."

If the teenager is mired in hopelessness or anxiety, another potentially helpful approach is to say, "All right, what's the very worst that could happen?"

Dr. Howard Newburger, a psychologist in Rye, New York, uses this approach in an exercise he calls "Flooding," and he reports that it has good results in many instances: "If a teenager is afraid to go to class because he might be called on to speak and then get up and say something stupid or wrong, you can piece together a fantasy of the very worst that could happen," says Dr. Newburger. "Let's say that the teenager gives an obviously wrong answer in class. Everyone laughs and jeers. The teacher is so overcome that she rushes from the classroom to tell the principal about the teen's incredibly stupid remark. The principal makes an announcement over the PA system for an immediate all-school assembly where the unfortunate student is asked to repeat his remark for the entire student body and faculty to hear. They all laugh and jeer at him for the rest of the day. By late afternoon, a TV news film crew arrives on the scene to capture his remark for the nightly news, and the next morning his dumb remark is a banner headline— accompanied by his most unflattering school picture—on the front page of the *New York Times*.

"Obviously, this fantasy is ridiculous, but when carried to an extreme like this, it helps to put things in perspective. The teen will realize that this can't happen and that any embarrassing situation he experiences won't come close to this catastrophe."

It also helps to work on bolstering your child's self-esteem, helping him or her feel good about himself as an intrinsically worthwhile human being. A number of teens with school phobia lack the self-esteem and confidence to tackle problems and challenges and, instead, feel overwhelmed by them.

INTERVENE WITH CARE

There is a fine line between constructively intervening in a problem situation (for example, a difficult teacher) as a necessary advocate for your child and undermining your child's self-esteem by taking over his problems and perhaps making them worse through your intervention. Before you make the decision to intervene, seek as much information as you can from your teenager and try active listening and problem solving together. If one teacher has a difficult, abrasive personality, it might be more useful if you listened with empathy to your teenager's complaints and then encouraged her to find ways to coexist with this difficult person. Learning to cope with someone who is demanding and perhaps a bit irrational can be a valuable life skill. On the other hand, if the teacher continues to be an overwhelming problem and is doing real harm—emotionally, academically or even physically—it may be best to step in and give your child a hand. Schedule a low-key, information-gathering conference with the teacher. If this proves unsatisfactory, talk with your child's counselor or with the principal.

Usually, you can help most by allowing your teen to fight her own battles— with your warm and constant support.

ENCOURAGE YOUR TEENAGER TO OVERCOME THE PHOBIA

Counseling and psychotherapy can be quite helpful to your teen in conquering school phobia. Family therapy, which may uncover and resolve some of the underlying conflicts that may contribute to your child's school phobia, is also a good idea. Don't encourage such behavior by allowing the child to stay home regularly or for long periods of time. This only reinforces the phobia and makes it more difficult than ever for the teenager to return to school. Your patience, support and firm encouragement for the child to attend school at least part of every day will help a great deal.

"For most school phobics, we try to get them out of the house and into a special school setting for a while," says educational psychologist Sarah Napier. "Or we get them in school for only two periods a day with the idea that they will gradually increase the number of class periods in time or participate in work experience programs. Our main goal is to get the teenager out of the house and doing something—however minimal it may be."

ENLIST THE AID OF YOUR CHILD'S TEACHERS

"When Rachel was having so much trouble with school phobia, I went to her guidance counselor and all her teachers and let them know about her problem," says Cynthia Bachman. "They were all wonderful to both Rachel and me. All said that this was not unusual, that they had seen the problem before in other students. That really surprised me. I had thought we were the only ones. Suddenly, I didn't feel that we were all alone—and that helped a lot."

In many cases, school officials and teachers are valuable allies and advocates and may guide you toward special programs and support services as well as lending much-needed support during this trying time.

13

Truancy and Other Serious School Problems

Although school phobics and truants both miss classes constantly and suffer from depression and myriad other family and emotional problems, there is a significant difference between the school phobic and the habitual truant. The phobic is afraid to go to school. The truant doesn't want to go and will not go to school for any number of reasons.

A report from the California Assembly Office of Research revealed that California's truancy and dropout rate among twelve- to seventeen-year-olds is about three times the national average. While pregnancy and marriage were cited as significant factors in truancy and school dropouts, reasons most often cited by students for truancy included dislike of or boredom with school, family or personal problems, academic problems, difficulties with social adjustment and the influence of friends.

"Some kids feel that school has nothing to offer and have friends who are also truant or who have dropped out," says Sarah Napier. "Some kids are overwhelmed by the pressures and expectations of school and simply can't cope."

Corbett Phibbs, a Westlake, California, family therapist who directs a special "T-Program" to help truant students and their families, feels that there is frequently a link between problems at home and trouble at school. In fact, he notes, trouble at school can be an early clue to masked conflicts within the family. "The actual causes of pain within a family system are almost never observable by the family members themselves," he says. "These problems are also rarely the ones the family believes they have. Often a child's destructive behavior has a very logical purpose, and in therapy I focus on teaching the family new ways to meet such purposes."

Control is a frequent source of family conflict, with school being one of the few areas of life where the adolescent feels he or she has some measure of control. Parents are relatively helpless in keeping a teenager from flunking or skipping classes. "This is a very effective way for the teenager to gain power, even if it is self-destructive in the long run," says Phibbs.

How You Can Help

What can you do if your teenager is truant or in continual trouble at school? There are a number of ways you can help—and get help.

BE OPEN TO ALL ALTERNATIVES

Although laws requiring school attendance up to a certain age vary by state, parents are usually notified and asked to cooperate in helping to keep an underage child in school after attendance has become a problem.

If your teenager is truant or disruptive in classes, there are a number of alternatives for help. You may find special help via school-based programs, through outside agencies and through private counseling or therapy.

Many school districts offer alternative or continuation programs that enable teens with attendance problems to stay in school and complete requirements for a high school diploma. Some of these special programs, which vary from state to state and district to district, include the following types:

Work-study programs: Work-study programs combine shortened academic class days with work experience carrying academic credit. Often this means that the students spend half a day in the classroom and half a day on the job.

Special classes: Alternative, night and special classes allow students to progress toward a diploma at an individualized pace. For the very depressed school-phobic teenager, this means temporary home teaching or a shortened school day, a lighter class load and lowered stress and expectations.

School furlough: School furlough programs give students academic credit for working, with no class attendance required for a specified amount of time.

Independent study programs: These are similar to furlough, work-study or alternative school programs. In 1976, for example, the California state legislature created an independent study program as an alternative to regular classroom study for students from kindergarten to twelfth grade. The major focus of the program was on high school dropouts or truants, but it has been utilized by students with psychological or medical problems and those with special career interests or talents in the arts or sports (for example, competitive figure skating, ballet, music or theater).

Early graduation: Early graduation opportunities offer students a chance to finish high school ahead of schedule and get out into the workforce or into special vocational programs or to go to college early.

CONTRACTING

Regular attendance at school is probably one of the major expectations you have for your teenager. You should make your teen aware of your expectations and establish firm guidelines.

Donna and Sam Wilson, for example, developed a contract with their fifteen-year-old daughter, Suzanne, to put a stop to her pattern of truancy. During a family meeting, Suzanne told her parents that she felt she had no say about how she spent her time, and she was convinced that her parents' expectation that she make top grades was unrealistic. Instead of fighting a futile battle to meet these expectations, and in an effort to get free, unstructured time of her own, Suzanne had been skipping classes several days a week.

As a result of this discussion, the Wilsons drew up a contract stating that as long as Suzanne took the responsibility to attend school regularly and do the best she could, her parents would not pressure her to make the honor roll and would allow her to structure her time as she pleased if homework and household chores got done. The arrangement has worked very well for them over the past year. "By lowering our expectations but stating clearly what we *did* expect, we ended up with more," says Donna Wilson. "Suzanne is going to school and doing just fine, and as a family, we have far fewer conflicts now."

DE-EMPHASIZE SCHOOL ATTENDANCE AS A CONTROL ISSUE

School is often the stage of adolescent acting out because it is one of the few areas where teenagers feel they have a fair amount of control, and they use this control to fight back with parents who may be overcontrolling them.

By making clear to your adolescent that school attendance is her responsibility and that she will have to face the consequences of not meeting this responsibility, you decrease the appeal of nonattendance at school as an acting-out alternative.

It is important *not* to take on the task of lying or covering up for your truant teenager. A number of parents do this against their better judgment because they hate to see their teens get into trouble with school authorities. However, such covering up simply reinforces the truant behavior and shelters the adolescent from its consequences.

It is more constructive to let your teen get a taste of trouble and learn from this experience. This does not mean, of course, that you should not be supportive and concerned when your teenager is troubled and having difficulties at school. It simply means that you will help most if you avoid assuming the role of accomplice to her truancy—by writing notes excusing her absences or by otherwise covering up and reinforcing her behavior.

In some instances, it is best to let your teenager work out school attendance problems with a third party while you stay out of the discussion altogether, giving up the control for this area of your child's life and handing it over to your child and a counselor. This is a good alternative if control is a volatile issue between you and your child.

TAKE AN INTEREST IN YOUR CHILD'S SCHOOL

In these days of two-career families or frantically busy single parents with many competing responsibilities, obligations and interests, parental involvement in school activities is on the wane. However, your interest and involvement in your child's school may help to rekindle your teen's own interest as well and gives the feeling that you consider him—and this area of his life—important.

Make an effort to attend school plays, sports events, parent-teacher conferences and open houses. Become involved in parental activities related to school. As an investment of your time, this can bring many rewards.

KNOW YOUR RIGHTS AND BE AN ADVOCATE FOR YOUR CHILD

By becoming involved, knowing your child's teachers and knowing your rights, you can help prevent serious school problems or you can help your child promptly if there is trouble.

"By cultivating good relationships within the school setting and by knowing your teenager's friends' parents, you can get feedback from others about early symptoms of trouble so that you can help your teenager before his problems reach the crisis stage," says special-education teacher Mary Ann Dan. "Some schools will give you feedback and some won't. It depends a great deal on the teachers. Some are very helpful. Also, when it comes to dealing with school bureaucracies, a kid may need a parent to troubleshoot."

Troubleshooting may mean having a low-key information-gathering conference with an allegedly troublesome teacher if problems with that class seem to be at the center of your teen's truancy, school phobia or serious depression. It may mean gaining access to your child's school records to get an erroneous, potentially harmful notation removed. It may mean meeting with your child's counselor, teachers and other school officials to determine the best alternatives when trouble develops.

A number of parents have difficulty dealing with school bureaucracy; they are possibly plagued by ghosts of their own academic pasts cautioning them not to make waves. You may be stalled and frustrated by indifference, hostility or bureaucratic clichés such as "That's not our policy" or "That's not the way we do things." Knowing the rules and your rights will make your advocacy easier and more effective.

"Find out how the school operates," suggests Ms. Dan. "Do they notify you after your child's third absence? Never? Would they be cooperative if you call in to check if your child is at school? Who might be a good in-school advocate for your child? Many parents assume that it is the child's guidance counselor, but this may not be the case. Counselors these days are overburdened. Your child's best advocate may be an especially interested, involved teacher who can help your child. Also, encourage your teen to tell you when he is in trouble. If there is a problem with one class and one teacher, your empathetic listening and gentle guidance—helping your child to see that some teachers do fall quite a bit short of the ideal but can be coped with—may be all your child needs. On the other hand, in serious matters you may be needed to troubleshoot. That's where knowing the school rules, who the good guys are and your rights as a parent come in handy."

Ms. Dan continues, "Know the law regarding class schedules, suspension and the like for your state. It's important for you to be knowledgeable and assertive enough to know what the *law*—as opposed to local school rules—says."

If your child is having problems at school, it's important to listen to feedback from teachers and school officials and consider their suggestions. "Some parents acknowledge that the child has a problem but want us to fix the child rather than seek help and work things out with the aid of a counselor," says Sarah Napier. "Others overreact to school problems or failures. I always try to reassure them by saying, 'Hey, your child is *not* bad. You just don't like some of his behavior.' If school personnel come to you with a problem, be willing to talk about it and what can be done."

Assuming a defensive attitude—refusing to hear negative feedback about your child, blaming others for your child's problems, defending your child relentlessly (even though you know that he did something wrong and/or has a problem)—can close off some vital sources of help and information. Listen to what you're hearing from teachers and school officials and weigh it carefully before springing to your child's defense. Sometimes the best way to help your child is to hear—and try to understand—the extent of his problems. This isn't easy. It can be painful, bringing feelings of guilt and inadequacy as a parent, feelings of fierce love and sadness and the desire to protect your troubled child, feelings that you and your child are misunderstood. Whether or not you ultimately agree with what you're hearing, listening carefully to feedback from your child's school will give you the information either to begin to work in concert with school officials to help your child or to frame an effective argument and/or advocacy campaign on your child's behalf.

Hopelessness and passivity are of no help to you or your child. Some parents, beleaguered by teenagers with continuing school problems, can't imagine that any alternative will help matters. "This 'Why bother?' attitude only reinforces the problem," says Sarah Napier. "Some kids say, 'My parents have written me off, so why bother to change?' But I believe that in most instances there *is* a solution to a teenager's problem with school. The solutions and changes may not be instantaneous, but they can make a difference. I tell distressed parents, 'We *can* make a change. It may not be a great one. It may not happen tomorrow. But at this point any change will help and it *can* happen.'"

Trouble at school may be, in one sense, a positive development when it functions as an early warning signal that all is not well with your teenager, enabling you to help her before the trouble and the pain escalate. If you are aware, informed, involved and open to all alternatives for help, school problems will provide you with an opportunity to assist your teenager early on and in a vital area of life. Offer your child your own special, caring help in dealing with the academic and social stressors so endemic to adolescent school experiences and you will enable your teenager to grow and develop resilience and independence—while ensuring a brighter future.

Part V

MEDICAL PROBLEMS AND TEENAGE DEPRESSION

14

When Your Child Has Depression-Linked Symptoms or Medical Conditions

Staci Pensak's gastrointestinal symptoms seemed to parallel her anxiety and depression over her family's move from Los Angeles to Yakima, Washington. "I felt like everyone hated me at first at my new school because I didn't fit in at all," says the fifteen-year-old sophomore. "Every school day, I had like these awful stomach cramps and pains. And I would get diarrhea every day at school, which was totally embarrassing, especially if I had to leave a class to go to the bathroom. At first I thought it was the yucky food in the school cafeteria, but it happens even if I bring my lunch. When my parents took me to a doctor, they were scared that I had some awful disease. But I had these tests and my doctor says it's irritable bowel syndrome, which is made worse by my bad feelings about school. I'm a little better since taking some medicine and trying some stress management stuff. It also helps that I'm getting used to my school and have a few friends now. But my parents are upset with me when I have stomach problems because they say it's all in my head. But I'm not making it up! It's real—believe me!"

At this time last year, Gina Lupi was slightly overweight and occasionally prone to cake, cookie and pretzel feasts. Then a gym teacher casually remarked that Gina would look terrific and be in great shape with a five- to ten-pound weight loss. So Gina started a diet with an important difference: She stuck to it. At first her parents were pleased. Then Gina began to subsist on two lettuce leaves and a pickle a day, and to exercise frenetically every minute she wasn't studying or sleeping. Finally, when she had shriveled down to seventy-eight pounds (while still insisting that she was a bit too heavy), her parents became genuinely alarmed. They took her to a physician, who recognized her symptoms immediately as signs of anorexia nervosa, an eating disorder characterized by compulsive self-starvation. While the disorder may involve a number of factors, depression can play a major role in the development and progression of the disease.

Frank Austin's diabetes was first diagnosed when he was ten. Once he and his parents adjusted to the dietary and lifestyle requirements that go along with successful management of the disease, things went smoothly— for a while. Now that Frank is fourteen, his diabetes and its management have become a central issue in family conflicts and in his growing depression. Frank accuses his parents of treating him like a kid when they try to help him manage his schedule of insulin injections, snacks and meals. And he fights back by refusing to keep on his schedule and by eating forbidden foods. His actions also show some evidence of denial—denial of the fact that his medical problem makes him a bit different in some respects. This fact is a very painful one for Frank. He wants to be one of the gang—to eat junk food, drink milk shakes and eat when he feels like it instead of when he has to, to be free of blood testing, insulin injections, doctor visits and parental hassles. He fears that the difference diabetes makes in his life will keep him from living a full and normal life forever. Frank was particularly distressed when he read in a magazine article that diabetes can be a factor in impotence. He wonders if his disease will keep him from having a normal sex life—or *any* sex life. But this concern isn't something he feels he can bring up with his parents or even his physician, and so his depression and sense of isolation are deepening.

Staci, Gina and Frank are only three of thousands of teenagers suffering from a combination of physical and emotional ills. The mind-body link is a fascinating one and is receiving an increasing amount of attention in medical circles these days. Researchers continue to examine the link between stress or other emotional problems, such as depression and anxiety, and physical illness, tracing susceptibility, disease progression and survival patterns in a variety of physical illnesses from the common cold to lupus and cancer.

One of the most famous studies on the correlation between stress and susceptibility to physical illness was conducted by Dr. Thomas H. Holmes

III, professor of psychiatry at the University of Washington. The study resulted in the Holmes-Rahe Scale, a stress-rating scale that assigns points to both positive and negative life changes (from a death in the family to marriage, starting or leaving school, taking a vacation or enjoying outstanding personal achievement). Dr. Holmes concluded that if a person scores 300 or more change points in a year, he has an 80 percent chance of experiencing a change of health. And since all change—both positive and negative—carries stress points, these points add up fast.

In a study at Stanford University Medical Center, Dr. Gordon Pulford, a clinical professor of pediatrics, developed a stress scale especially for teenagers, assigning 78 stress points for marriage (at such a young age), 108 points for the death of a parent, 70 for a parental divorce and 39 for either a romantic breakup or being rejected *or* accepted by the college of one's choice. Again, a total of 300 points or more is seen to be linked quite often with the development of physical problems.

In another study, this one by the Division of Adolescent Medicine at Montefiore Hospital and Medical Center in New York, physicians discovered that 30 percent of the teenagers coming into the adolescent clinic for treatment of physical complaints were also suffering from underlying depression, which was detected through special testing.

The mind-body connection between emotions and physical ailments is particularly strong and troublesome in adolescence. There are a number of reasons why this is so.

First, faced with the dramatic and rapid physical changes that puberty brings, teenagers are strongly focused on their bodies. "Being different or being in pain makes it particularly difficult for a teenager to cope," says Dr. Lonnie K. Zeltzer, director of Pediatric Pain Management at UCLA Medical Center. "Teenagers are so aware of their bodies and so worried about being normal. When they feel pain, they may panic and have a lot of anxiety about this being something serious, even fatal."

And defects, deviations, handicaps or physical illnesses can hit teenagers hard emotionally, often causing poor body image and depression.

Second, adolescence is a time of strong and conflicting emotions: love and anger, a growing need for independence coupled with a yearning to cling to and be protected by parents and strong new sexual urges countered by guilt, to name just a few. These conflicting feelings are stressful, often difficult to identify and impossible for some teens to express directly. So quite often the body does the speaking, signaling repressed feelings and conflicts through a variety of psychosomatic complaints.

These complaints are also a way of staying close and retaining a measure of dependence while growing toward adulthood and independence. "Being sick can be a binding thing that keeps the teenager tied to parents," says Dr. Marilyn Mehr. "And if illness is the only time the teenager receives attention and love from the parents, the body may signal what the mind is saying ('I need love!') via physical symptoms."

Third, the rapid growth that takes place in adolescence may cause physical and emotional depletion that can be a factor in depression.

The mind-body link shows itself in a number of ways. Depression or stress can trigger physical symptoms such as headaches, stomach pains, fatigue and sleep disorders, with the body expressing feelings and conflicts that the teen is unable to verbalize. Depression can be a factor, too, in causing or intensifying certain physical problems such as eating disorders (from anorexia nervosa to compulsive overeating) or asthma, lupus and other chronic disorders. It is also not uncommon for a physical condition such as diabetes, epilepsy, or scoliosis or a physical handicap to be a major factor in a teenager's depression.

Symptoms and Conditions That May Be Triggered or Intensified by Depression

PHYSICAL SYMPTOMS

The impact of depression and stress on your teenager's health may show in a number of ways. Have you noticed recently that your teenager has been:

- particularly susceptible to colds?
- suffering from more headaches than usual?
- listless, fatigued and sleeping a lot?
- unable to sleep at night?

- suffering from frequent diarrhea or alternating bouts of constipation and diarrhea?
- losing—or dramatically gaining—in appetite and weight?

If so, emotional conflicts may be a key factor. Some of the most frequently observed depression-linked physical symptoms include the following:

Fatigue: Maybe your previously alert and active teen has hit a slump and spends most of his or her time at home sleeping or lounging listlessly. Perhaps he complains of low energy, feelings of weakness and a sense of being tired all the time, no matter how much sleep he gets. And maybe your teen is completely immobilized by fatigue, unable to function in normal day-to-day ways. If so, depression is one of a number of possible causes to be considered.

"I've had a number of teenagers come in to see me complaining of fatigue and excessive sleeping," says Dr. Charles Wibbelsman. "They often come in saying, 'I think I have mono' or 'I must be anemic.' That could be, but often the teenager doesn't have any underlying medical problem. Yet he is tired all the time and sleeps twelve to fourteen hours a day. When a physical disease is not present, this fatigue could well be a sign of underlying depression."

Sleep disorders: Depression can disturb sleep patterns in people of all ages, but it shows up in special ways among depressed teens. While a depressed adult may fall asleep at night with difficulty or may be plagued by early awakening in predawn hours, unable to get back to sleep, a depressed teenager usually suffers from insomnia.

"A change of sleep patterns is a very common sign of depression in teenagers," says Dr. Richard MacKenzie. "Some teens (I've noticed this particularly in teenagers who are also suffering from anorexia nervosa) stay up all night and then sleep during the day."

Vague aches and pains: The depressed teenager may experience painful emotions through physical discomfort, complaining of annoying pain in a number of body areas. "Low back pain, in particular, may be tied to depression," Dr. MacKenzie observes.

Stomach pains and disorders: "The gastrointestinal tract, most notably the stomach and intestines, is quite easily affected by the emotions," says Dr. Wibbelsman. "It may take a stomachache, diarrhea or more alarming symptoms to point out to parents just how tense, depressed, frightened or angry the teenager is feeling."

Gastritis, the secretion of excess acid in the stomach, can occur as the result of tension and anxiety. This excess acid begins to digest the stomach lining, causing pain and heartburn, and may lead to an ulcer.

Diarrhea can be another sign of emotional distress. "We see this quite often around exam times when teens are nervous about school performance," says Dr. Wibbelsman. "This condition can come from anxiety or poor diet and frequently is due to a combination of the two."

Another condition with a possible link to emotions is colitis or irritable bowel syndrome (IBS). It may be signaled by alternating bouts of diarrhea and constipation, pain, nausea, heartburn and a feeling of faintness. Those most at risk for this disorder are depressed, or they have a childhood history of physical or sexual abuse, have experienced the loss of one or both parents during childhood, have high levels of stress with low levels of support from family or friends and have a possible genetic predisposition to the disorder.

Ulcerative colitis, a potentially serious condition found primarily in young people, occurs when ulcers develop in the colon, and the walls of the colon become inflamed and diseased. Symptoms of ulcerative colitis include cramps, bloody stools, diarrhea and painless rectal bleeding. A number of factors contribute to the development of this disease, but emotional stresses—depression and anxiety among them—play a major role in causing or aggravating this disease.

Headaches: Headaches are very common among depressed teenagers, especially teenage girls. "This may be because girls are particularly prone to internalize their feelings, to hold in their anger and depression," says Dr. Mehr.

Dr. Merilee Oaks concurs, noting that she sees headaches most often in Latino teenagers. "They have a lot of psychosomatic symptoms in connection with anger and depression," she says. "These girls are caught in a cultural conflict. They are growing up in the freedom of the American culture while living in families with parents and grandparents whose values are rooted in a quite different culture. These girls don't know how to fight back or express themselves because their families' cultural mores say that you must not argue with elders. So they have a lot of headaches. I've seen even *daily* migraines among these girls. Underlying these headaches is a lot of anger and depression about being in a situation where the teen sees no way out until adulthood."

While headaches come from a number of physical causes, including sinus infections, dental problems, allergies, high blood pressure, skipping a meal, smoking too much and, rarely, a brain tumor, chronic headaches often result from a combination of physical and psychological factors. Feelings, including depression, can be involved in a number of different kinds of headaches—including tension and psychogenic or migraine headaches.

Tension headaches, stemming most often from anxiety and tense shoulder and neck muscles, are signaled by throbbing pain felt at the front or sides of the skull. A tension headache is often relieved by aspirin or other over-the-counter painkillers and rest.

Psychogenic headaches, which involve tense muscles in the face, head and neck, often stem from depression and feel like a tight band circling the head. These headaches tend to strike early in the morning and are usually seen in combination with other signs of depression such as sleep disorders. Pain relievers, emotional support and professional counseling may be needed in order to combat these headaches.

Migraine headaches (also called vascular headaches) are severe and may be triggered by:

• hormonal changes: They usually occur for the first time in girls around the time of puberty and may occur more frequently around the time of menstruation.
• environmental factors: smoke-filled rooms, bright sunlight, heavy traffic and gasoline fumes and the like.
• lifestyle and eating habits: irregular sleep patterns; eating foods such as cheese, lima beans, Chinese food with MSG and chocolate or drinking alcohol, which may stimulate the affected blood vessels.
• emotional stress: especially when caused by repressed anger, frustration and depression.

In a 1990 study comparing 162 young adults with migraines with the same number of peers who did not have migraines, researchers found that severe depression, anxiety and insomnia were much more common in the young people who had migraine headaches. The headaches were not a factor in causing these emotional states, but rather were most likely to occur in those who had some emotional upheavals in their lives.

There are a number of different kinds of migraine headaches. The two most common are classic and common migraines. In the classic variety, the victim experiences an aura—flashing lights or colors or spots before the eyes—or mood changes before the headache's pain strikes. In common migraines, the aura may not be present, but the characteristic migraine symptoms are there: pain on one side of the head, throbbing initially and then becoming steady and unrelenting; sensitivity to light and noise; nausea and, in some cases, dizziness and loss of balance.

Migraine headaches may be treated in a number of ways, often with a combination of prescription painkillers, dietary and lifestyle changes, biofeedback and stress management techniques and perhaps psychotherapy to enable the teen to express rather than repress feelings.

Why Do Teens Express Emotional Pain with Physical Symptoms?

Why do teens so often use their bodies to express the emotional pain and conflicts they feel? It may be because physical ills are often viewed with more importance than emotional pain by parents, teachers or even the teens themselves.

"It's much easier for kids to ask for medical care than for psychological help," says Dr. Marilyn Mehr. "They often have a great fear of being crazy or of being *thought* to be crazy."

The reactions of adults to these physical signals can be crucial in helping the teenager feel better or in making him feel worse. Some of the mistakes that parents make are typical of the reactions that Ed and Marilyn Hartman had to the recurring headaches and stomach pains that their daughter Dana has suffered for the past six months.

Initially concerned, they took her to the family doctor for a checkup. When medical tests failed to detect any organic causes for Dana's distress, the physician, an older man with little interest in teenagers, told her parents,

"It's psychological, part of being a teenager. I guess you'll all just have to bear with it until Dana grows up a little."

Now Ed and Marilyn discount Dana's symptoms when they occur—either ignoring her complaints or telling her to grow up and stop whining and being such a hypochondriac. But Dana's body isn't listening. She still suffers real physical pain and deepening emotional pain, including depression, a growing sense of isolation and hopelessness.

"Silence, lecturing or labeling doesn't make the pain go away," says Dr. Zeltzer. "I particularly dislike the term *hypochondriac* because it is so often misused as a label to mean 'faker.' I see many young people with stress-induced symptoms like chest and back pains, stomachaches, headaches and fatigue stemming from depression. I don't think for a minute that they're faking anything. Their pain and problems are real!"

"I cringe when I hear someone say, 'It's *just* psychosomatic pain,'" adds Dr. Mehr. "The implication is that if it's psychosomatic, it isn't real. But of course the pain we see *is* real, both emotionally and physically."

Dr. Zeltzer points out that physical pain has many different causes. "When someone suffers pain, it may mean a disease like hepatitis, or depression over the loss of a love," she says. "Pain is a message. It is the body's way of signaling that something troubling is going on. The whole process of dealing with pain is to work with the person to help decode this message. Why is the pain there? What is going on? One person may have the flu, another may be depressed."

How You Can Help

There are a number of ways that you can help if your teenager is having physical symptoms that are psychosomatic.

WATCH FOR CHANGES IN YOUR TEEN'S HEALTH

Be aware of any changes in your teenager's health patterns or any troublesome physical symptoms. If these persist, mention your observations and your concern to your teenager. Encourage him or her to talk about how she is feeling, physically or emotionally.

DON'T AUTOMATICALLY REJECT THE REALITY OF SYMPTOMS

Don't dismiss symptoms with remarks such as "It's probably just in your head" or "Don't be such a baby" or "Just tough it out and it will go away." Pain is a valuable signal and should not be ignored or minimized. If a teenager needs to express emotional conflicts through physical distress, this is an important clue to a communication problem that exists within your family.

SEEK PROFESSIONAL HELP

Encourage your teenager to seek competent medical help and see that she gets it. Unless your teenager has a good and open relationship with the family doctor, consider getting a referral to a pediatrician or internist who specializes in adolescent medicine and who has special talent and training in communicating with and caring for teenagers. A doctor who knows how to listen and respond to a teenager's feelings and complaints and who will take the time to do so can be a great asset to your child's emotional and physical health.

A physical examination is vital, too, to make sure that the symptoms actually are emotionally linked and not due to a physical disorder. When the probable cause of the teen's distress is pinpointed, he is in a better position to receive appropriate help.

Medical help may be the most acceptable alternative, maybe the only one your teen will go along with at this time. "Many teens are resistant to mental-health care," says Dr. Richard Brown. "But they may go to a physician for a health checkup. If this physician is also sensitive to feelings and is good with adolescents, this kind of help is most valuable. The doctor checks the teen to eliminate the possibility of disease and makes an assessment of the teenager's complete health, including psychosocial development. If seeking professional help is approached from the standpoint of getting a health-care checkup—at least initially—this may be more acceptable to the teenager."

BE GENTLE WITH YOUR TROUBLED TEEN

If your teenager does have psychosomatic symptoms, be gentle with him. Don't label him as a malingerer, a baby or a troublemaker. It is much more constructive to validate the pain, saying, in effect, "I know you're hurting, and I want to help you in any way I can." Give time, attention and expressions of love to your child not only when he is sick or in pain but also at times when he is feeling well, too. Some parents unwittingly reward and reinforce sickly behavior by taking time to say "I love you" or "I care about you" only when their children are ill.

SEEK FAMILY COUNSELING IF MAJOR TENSIONS EXIST

If there are tensions within your family, try to get family counseling to find ways to change your own behavior and take the risk of communicating with each other. If you reduce some of these tensions and start to get feelings out into the open and learn to communicate more effectively, you will find that your child's symptoms may start to diminish. Some families are able to do this on their own, but many need extra help from a counseling professional. It's important to be open to this option if your family seems to be in trouble.

Preexisting Medical Conditions

Some medical conditions, while not caused by emotional conflicts, are adversely affected by such problems.

"We find that a lupus flare-up, for example, can be precipitated by emotional factors," says Dr. Merilee Oaks. "Also, asthma gets worse with emotional stress."

Because of the strong mind-body connection among many teens with severe asthma, some physicians treat these young people with a combination of drugs, psychotherapy and family counseling. In especially severe cases the asthma victim may have to live away from home for a while.

In the same way, emotional issues can cause difficulties with chronic medical conditions such as diabetes or epilepsy when a teen fails to follow an essential medical regimen because of denial, depression or rebellion.

Other medical conditions—colitis, ulcerative colitis, ulcers and migraine headaches—occur as the result of many factors, but are aggravated by emotional upsets.

How You Can Help

CONSULT YOUR PHYSICIAN

Check with your child's physician for reassurance and supportive care. If the physician is not supportive of your child's emotional as well as physical needs, it is time to search for another doctor or for counseling to supplement your child's medical care and to ease the stressors in his life, teaching him new ways of coping with the inevitable ups and downs.

TELL YOUR TEEN THAT YOU CARE

Communicate the fact that you care and that while the teen has primary responsibility for health maintenance, you're concerned and willing to help. Many parents assume that their teens know they care and will help. Never assume anything. Always try to make your loving, caring feelings clear to your child, but don't try to take over the problem.

COMMUNICATE WITH YOUR TEEN
ABOUT THE PROBLEM

Explore ways of dealing with stress and depression with your teenager. Approach this not as a lecture but as a dialogue, an idea-sharing session to help each other find more constructive ways to cope with tensions or troubling feelings. Here are some possible stress reducers that you might bring up in the discussion:

• Take the risk of talking openly instead of repressing feelings.

• Reassure your teen that expressing anger, needs, frustration and the like will not result in rejection. Then be true to your word, resolving to listen even when you don't like what you're hearing.

• Talk about expectations: the expectations you have for yourself and for each other—and how these can hurt when they're unrealistic. Sort out the realistic from the unrealistic—from both viewpoints—and discuss these with an open mind.

• Start a physical exercise regimen, with a physician's approval. Carefully chosen physical exercise reduces both tension and depression and does wonderful things for the body. If your teenager is reluctant to exercise, make it a joint effort—a shared time of self-renewal stressing companionship, not competition. This can go a long way toward reducing stress for both or all of you!

15

Depression and Eating Disorders

Eating disorders reflect myriad painful issues in a teenager's life. While a teen with mild temporary depression may lose his or her appetite for a few days, the problem can be much more severe in teenagers with serious depression and other emotional issues.

"The eating disorders that are linked with depression cover quite a wide range," says Dr. Donald McKnew. "The teenager may have poor appetite and weight loss or engage in compulsive overeating and experience a considerable weight gain."

Dr. Richard MacKenzie observed that "an eating disorder represents a teenager's attempt to gain some control by engaging in a behavior which cannot be regulated by another person. But often this is carried to an extreme."

Extreme conditions, such as anorexia nervosa or bulimia nervosa on the one hand, and compulsive eating and obesity on the other, may occur in conjunction with depression. Even if your depressed teenager is not experiencing these extremes of behavior, the discussion of them, along with general tips for helping, may give you some ideas for coping constructively with mild as well as severe eating disorders.

Eating Disorders: What Are They?

To begin with, from a clinical standpoint only anorexia nervosa and bulimia nervosa are considered to be eating disorders. Compulsive overeating and obesity or "fear of obesity" syndrome (which causes a young girl to diet stringently), without signs of the two clinically recognized eating disorders, may be viewed as problematic behaviors but are not, clinically, considered to be eating disorders. But, as most of us know, they can both reflect and cause a great deal of pain in a young person's life.

ANOREXIA NERVOSA

This is a serious psychosomatic disorder that afflicts primarily females (only about 4 percent of victims are male) and that involves compulsive dieting and starvation. It may be caused by a variety of emotional as well as physical factors.

Those with anorexia nervosa avoid food (even though they may be obsessed with preparing food for others); exercise compulsively; have a distorted body image of themselves as fat even when they have assumed skeletal proportions; refuse to maintain the minimum healthy body weight for their age, height and build; and experience amenorrhea (cessation of menstrual periods). They may also experience hair loss, low body temperature and dangerously low blood pressure.

Historically physicians and mental-health professionals have identified certain personality and family characteristics that occur with great frequency in those with anorexia. Victims are usually high-achieving, parent-pleasing girls from middle-class or affluent families.

"They are usually the jewels of their family, the until-now-problem-free children," says Dr. Richard MacKenzie, who has treated numerous teens with eating disorders over the years at Children's Hospital, Los Angeles. "The teenager has high expectations of herself and doesn't want to let her parents down."

There is usually a constellation of problems and issues simmering below the surface of this seemingly perfect child. Quite often another child in the family has had serious problems or the parents may have marital problems. There may be disturbances, too, in family relationships that make it more difficult than usual for the girl to achieve her developmental task of growing away from the parents: She and her mother often share a mutual dependency, and quite often the father doles out his love sparingly or conditionally, depending on the girl's achievements.

"Quite often there is a sort of Pygmalion relationship between father and daughter," says Dr. Robert Anderson of Columbia University Student Health Center. "The girl wants to be like the woman her father likes and she lives in accord with her father's wishes."

Underneath, this perfect daughter may carry a great deal of depression. "Major depression and dysthymia are two significant elements in eating disorders," says Dr. Roger Tonkin, who has conducted considerable research on the emotional factors of eating disorders. "In anorexia especially, the incidence of major depression is very high."

In recent years experts have also examined possible physical reasons why some girls—and not others—suffer from anorexia nervosa. A study at the National Institute of Mental Health found that a group of women with anorexia had an unusual amount of brain secretions of a hormone called vasopressin, which regulates the body's water balance. Researchers theorize that this unusual hormonal response could be a factor in tipping the balance between an ordinary diet and compulsive starvation. Dr. Philip Gold, the primary researcher in the study, believes that while perfectionism may be the driving factor at the beginning of a girl's quest for thinness, certain biological changes that take place when she drops below a certain weight—including changes in levels of vasopressin—cause the victim to become compulsive and irrational in her dieting efforts.

Researchers at Wayne State University found that those with anorexia may be physically addicted to dieting. When food intake drops, the release of brain opioids causes the dieter to experience a pleasant high. With anorexia, this high may be so intense that victims get addicted to it and don't want to lose this feeling by eating.

The health—even life—risks of anorexia nervosa are considerable. Between 5 and 15 percent of all victims die from complications of the disorder, and surviving victims often suffer from severe malnutrition, dangerously low blood pressure, cardiac arrhythmias (irregular heartbeats), osteoporosis and general poor health.

BULIMIA NERVOSA

Bulimia is a somewhat more common eating disorder than anorexia, affecting four out of every 100 women between the ages of seventeen and twenty-five.

Those with bulimia are usually normal weight or just slightly overweight and seek to control weight by self-induced vomiting and laxative abuse. Additionally, a recent study at the University of Minnesota found that some bulimics overuse saunas in order to shed water weight. In addition to purging behaviors, bulimics have regular food binges during which they may consume large quantities of food and then vomit immediately to keep from gaining weight.

While bulimics also tend to be overachieving females with low self-esteem and higher than usual levels of depression and also come from upper-middle-class homes, they differ from anorexics in several important ways. Bulimics are more likely to have experienced childhood physical or sexual abuse and to have continued to have abusive relationships into young adulthood. They are more likely to engage in alcohol or drug abuse and to come from families in which there are addictive disorders. Some studies show that up to 75 percent of bulimics have suffered from major depression.

There are also some recent findings that the development of bulimia may have a physical basis. A study at the National Institute of Mental Health found that bulimics, as well as anorexics, have excessive levels of the brain hormone vasopressin. Another NIMH study, in conjunction with Duke University, found that many women with bulimia fail to secrete normal levels of the hormone cholecystokinin, which produces a feeling of fullness after a meal. Another study, this one at the University of Pittsburgh, found that a low level of serotonin in the brain can be a factor in binge eating. (Serotonin is neurotransmitter, low levels of which can also be a factor in depression.)

Like anorexia, bulimia is a complex and dangerous disorder with potentially life-threatening consequences. Most deaths occur as the result of rupture of the esophagus from vomiting or from ipecac poisoning or cardiac arrest, especially common among those who use and abuse laxatives or diuretics.

What Are the Common Eating Problems?

Eating problems that fall short of clinical classification but that can be the cause or the symptom of significant problems for teenagers include fear-of-obesity syndrome and compulsive overeating/obesity.

FEAR-OF-OBESITY SYNDROME

Much of the behavior in this syndrome looks like anorexia but is not as intense. The teen may avoid food, diet stringently and think she's fat when she's not. But she is less likely to have the same constellation of emotional problems or the same dramatic weight loss as the teen with anorexia.

There is always the danger, however, that this behavior can evolve into anorexia or bulimia, as well as interfere with a girl's growth and development.

COMPULSIVE OVEREATING/OBESITY

This can be a very painful problem for teens and their families. Teens who have an overeating problem tend to eat when not hungry, eat normally at mealtimes but binge in secret and overeat when angry, upset or nervous *or* to celebrate a happy event. They also tend to react with overeating behavior when reminded, or nagged, about their weight.

Some adolescents overeat to anesthetize feelings of fear, anxiety and anger, as well as use food as a tranquilizer in times of positive or negative stress.

In his research on obese patients eating in response to stress, Dr. Neil Solomon of Johns Hopkins Medical School has noted that very often the stress eater feels underlying hostility toward some person or situation but would rather eat than voice such hostilities.

Some teens take refuge in their fat in order to avoid romantic or sexual involvements and to postpone decisions about their sexuality. This is especially true for a teenager who has experienced sexual trauma at an early age.

Other teens who are depressed, bored and losing interest in everything turn to food to fill the void in their lives. And some use food, and being overweight, as a means of rebellion. In this instance, compulsive eating is much like anorexia, with the teenager struggling to seize control of her life the only way she knows how. Teens whose parents put a high premium on good looks, physical fitness or popularity are especially prone to this type of rebellion.

Dr. Johanna T. Dwyer studied a group of obese young women at Harvard University and discovered that many of them had mothers who pushed them to succeed at everything and who talked about thinness as some kind of moral virtue and being fat as the worst possible fate. These young women fought back by making their mothers' vision of the worst possible fate a reality.

"A power struggle is the basis of much adolescent obesity," says Dr. Merilee Oaks. "Obesity and sexuality are two areas where the teen can act out, saying, in effect, 'I own my body and there's nothing you can do about it.'"

Overeating may also be an expression of low self-esteem.

"Overeating is a way of not caring about oneself," says Dr. Richard MacKenzie. "The obese teenager is saying, in effect, 'I'm not worthwhile. Why should I care about myself?'"

The price that adolescents pay for expressing their feelings through overeating and obesity is high. The short-term price may be ridicule and exclusion by peers, as well as discrimination from employers and, in some instances, from college admissions officials. The long-term price may be even higher: Some 80 percent of obese adolescents become obese adults and are at high risk for life-threatening cardiovascular disease, adult-onset diabetes and some forms of cancer. Recent studies have found that boys who are obese in adolescence are at highest risk for medical problems as adults.

Who Is Most at Risk for Eating Disorders?

Victims of these official or unofficial eating disorders are overwhelmingly female—in part, at least, because females in our society are judged more stringently by looks and weight than are males. Especially in the past decade or so, the ideal female figure, represented by fashion models and actresses, has shrunk from the curvaceousness of Marilyn Monroe to a tall, slender, asexual ideal that is not achievable by most girls or women. It is interesting to note that only about 4 percent of those with anorexia nervosa are male, and of those, many participate in sports—such as wrestling or gymnastics—in which weight is a major consideration.

Young women most at risk for eating disorders or problems are those who reached physical maturity earlier than peers. Other high risks for eating disorders include teens who come from a family in which weight is an issue. Here, parents may have a weight problem or put a great value on slimness. And teens with authoritarian parents or those with substance-abusing parents are also a high risk for eating disorders.

How You Can Help

IF YOUR TEEN HAS AN EATING DISORDER SUCH AS ANOREXIA OR BULIMIA

• *Get immediate medical help.* The sooner your teenager gets treatment, the better.

Anorexia is usually treated with a combination of medical treatments (quite often inpatient hospitalization for a time) and individual and family therapy. Family therapy has been found to be especially useful for young adolescents, while older adolescents and young adults do best with individual therapy.

The prognosis for full recovery without serious health consequences is best when treatment starts *before* extreme weight loss occurs.

There are no fast and easy ways to treat anorexia. Some of the most successful treatment programs combine medical and psychological treatment in both inpatient and outpatient settings. Quite often at the beginning of treatment the teen is hospitalized (in order to get her into a controlled, therapeutic atmosphere and away from family tensions) with weight gain—not food intake—as a major goal.

Drug treatment for anorexia shows some promise, though experts emphasize that the disorder is too complex to be treated by drugs alone. Opioid inhibitors, a class of drugs that block the action of pleasure-causing brain opioids and help to break an anorexic's addiction to dieting, show particular promise. A review of several recent studies shows that 75 percent of patients treated with the drug Naltrexone gained a healthy amount of weight.

Bulimia also requires expert medical and psychological intervention. Some patients have improved after taking antidepressant medications such as monoamine-oxidase inhibitors, but some physicians hesitate to prescribe these drugs to severely depressed teens, who may commit suicide by taking an overdose of this powerful medication, or to patients whose persistent self-induced vomiting may diminish the effectiveness of the drug. Researchers hope that the continued development of drugs that affect serotonin levels in the brain may offer future help to those with bulimia, but many caution that drug treatment may lead to improvement but that total recovery depends on a multifaceted approach to treatment, with psychotherapy as a crucial element.

Close medical monitoring—even once the patient seems to have recovered from anorexia or bulimia—is crucial. The death of singer Karen Carpenter occurred when she was eating again and seemed to be recovering after a long struggle with anorexia. In a review of medical literature, Dr. Iris Litt and Dr. Barbara Palla of Stanford University found that anorexia- or bulimia-associated deaths occurred not only in the initial stages of treatment but also during recovery. In their own study at Stanford, Drs. Litt and Palla found that more than half of recovering anorexic patients and 22 percent of bulimic patients required hospitalization for medical reasons during the study period. They noted that "adolescent patients with anorexia nervosa and bulimia are physiologically unstable and at risk of dying."

So attempts at self-help, at psychotherapy alone or treatment by a physician not familiar with the treatment and risks of these serious eating disorders can be futile—even fatal.

• *De-emphasize the whole issue of eating.* It is important to de-emphasize control issues and emphasize personal responsibility in treatment. Let the physician, the psychotherapist and your teenager handle the problem. Compliment your teen on weight gains, emphasizing her new glow of health.

Watch your own behavior carefully to identify ways you may be contributing to the problem or sabotaging treatment. It is vital not to argue with, nag or lecture your teen or to attempt to take over or solve her problems for her. Control is a major issue in many eating disorders, and the more you try to superimpose your views and convictions in this area, the more serious and stubborn the battle will become.

• *Realize that there are no quick cures.* Treatment of these eating disorders takes a great deal of time and patience. Habits are hard to break, and depression may linger for a time. You may also notice that your teen may be less inclined to be perfect and more likely to voice negative feelings or get into direct conflicts as treatment progresses. As unsettling as these developments may be, they *are* signs of progress and yet another reason why the family as a whole needs to be in therapy with the adolescent. The change in one family member can trigger changes in the whole family system, and a supportive mental-health professional can be a great help to all of you.

IF YOUR TEEN HAS AN EATING PROBLEM SUCH AS COMPULSIVE OVEREATING

• *Get medical help and advice.* If your teen is suffering from fear-of-obesity syndrome, check with your physician about the availability of nutritional or behavioral counseling. If your adolescent is obese, his physician may be able to supervise a well-balanced eating plan or make a referral to a nutritionist-supervised regimen or to a program such as Shapedown or Weight Watchers. Treatment of obesity and compulsive-eating problems work best when parents step back and let the teen work with a medical or mental-health professional. But find out what the options are *before* involving your teen in the process.

• *Communicate your concern in a nonjudgmental way.* It's temptation when your teen is overeating and gaining weight to respond with anger, frustration and blunt observations such as: "If you don't stop eating like that, you'll weigh over three hundred pounds!" or "Do you realize how terrible you look?" or "Why can't you just control yourself? You're only making things worse!"

Such comments set the stage for a real control battle. It is more constructive to express concern and ask for some feedback from your teen, confronting him or her gently with your own observations and then asking what his or her feelings are.

"If your child hasn't mentioned weight as a problem or doesn't seem disturbed by it, you might make the observation: 'It looks to me like you're gaining weight. Does this bother you?'" suggests Dr. Merilee Oaks. "If the teen says, 'Yes,' you might then ask, 'Would you like help?' and then, with an affirmative answer, you might take the teen to a doctor and seek other resources as well. If the teenager says, 'No. It isn't a problem for me,' then express your own emotion, 'I worry about you,' and encourage the teenager to check with his or her physician, letting the doctor and teen discuss and deal with the possible problem."

In talking with your teen, don't be negative and say that he or she is bad or ugly, or should be ashamed of himself. Accent the positive: the importance of being as healthy and attractive as possible now and learning healthy eating habits early in life to prevent more serious problems later.

If your teen gets angry and refuses to discuss the matter, don't push. He may not be ready to tackle the weight problem or may feel the need to reject any ideas you present. This doesn't mean that you haven't been heard or that the teenager will never be motivated to lose weight. It may help to acknowledge your teen's reluctance to talk about this issue right now and let him know that you are ready to listen and help at any time. Then keep to your word.

• *De-emphasize control and emphasize responsibility.* To keep the issue of control from interfering with your teen's weight loss or habit-control progress, don't nag your child to stay on a diet, monitor food intake or weight loss or play detective. If you see him eating something decidedly inadvisable, bite your tongue, if necessary, to keep from asking, "Is *that* on your diet?" or saying, "You *know* you shouldn't be eating that." The teen knows and may be experiencing a bout of self-sabotage or testing your resolve. If you don't get hooked into old reaction patterns, the power of overeating as a means of re-bellion will be decreased. Communicate the concept "It's your body and your choice what you feed it" to diffuse the power of such rebellion.

• *Be aware of your own sabotaging behavior.* Even though on a conscious level you want very much for your teenager to lose weight, you may have subconscious fears about the changes that significant weight loss will bring. You may have hidden feelings of jealousy or competitiveness as your teenager begins to look more attractive. You may fear change as your child becomes more assertive, more self-confident and less dependent on you. Such feelings are not bad or unusual, but it is essential to be aware of them in order to mod-ify your own behavior. Are you sabotaging your teen's weight-loss program? You may be if:

you use food as a reward even now. Urging a high-fat favorite treat on him "just this once" as a reward or a gesture of love can sabotage his efforts and reinforce the old "food as reward, pacifier, etc." form of behavior. Find other ways to express your love and offer rewards.

you keep junk food around the house "for the family." Nobody needs junk food. See your teen's weight-loss efforts as an opportunity for the whole family to eat in a healthy way. Low-fat meals and lots of fruits and vegetables will be beneficial to everyone.

you make a weight-loss regimen seem like penance and treat your teen differently. Those who have the best results with losing weight and keeping it off are those who revise their eating habits permanently. Diets don't work—and the mentality of being on or off a diet leads to health-threatening yo-yo weight loss/gain patterns. Your teen isn't bad or morally corrupt for being obese, and weight loss isn't penance; it's a wise and healthy decision and, ideally, the beginning of a lifetime of healthy eating.

you give your teen attention only when he fails. This only reinforces neg-ative behavior. Praise him for trying, for all the effort that weight loss takes, not for the end result. If your adolescent has a great deal of weight to lose, it will take some time before the results are evident. Praise your teenager for his strength and resolve, one day at a time. Let him know that you know how difficult it is and how much you admire his efforts. Let him know, most of all, that your love is not contingent on how much or how little he weighs.

• *Encourage more physical activity.* Help your teen find fun and interesting activities that involve exercise. Invest in a good exercise bicycle or cross-country ski machine if your teen is too embarrassed to exercise in public. If it would be helpful, join him in some exercise or activity such as walking, cycling or swimming as a way of giving time, attention and continuing encouragement.

CHAPTER

16

When Being Different Brings On Depression

Bob Allen is fourteen but looks several years younger. He is mortified over his short stature and lack of physical development, especially when he compares himself to his peers in the locker room or when classmates tease him about being short. He is wondering when, if ever, he'll finally grow up to look like everyone else.

Jessica Dunning, on the other hand, is embarrassed about her height: She's five feet eight inches tall at the age of thirteen and towers over most of the boys in her class.

Mike Swanson has been depressed lately because he feels that his epilepsy will make him even more different from his friends as he grows older. He is already dreading next year, when the other kids in his class will be getting their driver's licenses and he won't.

And Frank Austin, the young diabetic whose story appeared at the beginning of Chapter 15, finds a lot of pain in following or not following the strict regimen that his medical condition requires, a regimen he feels sets him apart from his friends and classmates.

Being different because of circumstances beyond one's control—because of late development, a chronic illness or a temporary or permanent handicap—is especially painful for the body-conscious teenager. Being different or *feeling* intrinsically different because of a physical problem can lead to poor body image, low self-esteem and depression.

"We see a great deal of depression in chronically ill adolescents," says Dr. Richard MacKenzie. "They feel different and bad about themselves because of this. They feel that their parents don't trust them. Also, the illness holds them back in the developmental process of emancipation from the family, and this causes depression as their self-esteem plummets."

How You Can Help

While you may not be able to change your child's physical problems, you can help to change his or her feelings and self-perceptions.

IF YOUR TEENAGER IS A LATE DEVELOPER

A medical checkup may reassure everyone that all is well, or if there is a problem, it may be a step toward getting help. In many instances late development is genetic. If you or your spouse happened to be a late bloomer, share your feelings and experiences with your child—not by minimizing the pain of being different right now, but by reassuring your child that he or she *will* develop and that there is a wide range of normal development in the teen years.

IF YOUR TEENAGER IS UNUSUALLY TALL OR SHORT

Listen to your teen's feelings about height and explore ways to cope and compensate. If, for example, your junior high–age daughter is worried about being taller than many boys in her class, it's quite possible that most of them will catch up with and even surpass her in height in a year or two and that she will not always be so different.

If your son or daughter is past the age of puberty, is in the mid-to-late teens and is still significantly shorter or taller than peers, don't keep saying, "You'll grow!" or "They'll grow and catch up with you." It's important not to give your teen the idea that it's not normal to be as he or she is. The concepts that men *must* be taller than women or that women must physically look up to men are arbitrary, culturally imposed traditions—ones that are certainly worth questioning. In the past and even in the present, these traditions have prevented many loving, fulfilling relationships from happening and, more important, have caused many men and women to feel terrible about themselves. It is difficult to say, especially to a self-conscious teen, that cultural mores don't matter at all. But it helps to start exploring them with your teen, raising the question "Why must we meet certain culturally imposed height standards if being a certain stature is normal for you?"

Help your tall or short teen accept and adjust to his or her body by pursuing special physical activities. Dance or modeling classes may help a tall girl feel less awkward and more graceful. Sports such as gymnastics, figure skating or running, and noncompetitive but stamina-building activities such as dancing or weight training, may help enhance your short or tall teen's body image considerably.

FIND WAYS TO HELP PHYSICALLY HANDICAPPED TEENS FEEL MORE ATTRACTIVE

Good grooming habits, attractive hairstyles and flattering, well-designed clothes will help the disabled teenager acquire a more positive body image. Of course, personality and skill compensations are also crucial, but for the body-conscious teen, being as attractive as possible is an important step toward feeling more normal and less depressed and different. Encourage your teenager to take an interest in enhancing physical strong points instead of taking a "Why bother?" attitude.

PUT RESPONSIBILITY FOR MANAGEMENT OF A CHRONIC DISEASE ON THE TEENAGER

This is especially important in chronic conditions such as diabetes and epilepsy in which lifelong responsibility is an important factor in successful health maintenance. When possible, keep management issues between your teenager and the physician so that the teen gets practice in taking responsibility and will not be as tempted to rebel against your authority by refusing to comply with disease treatment and management routines. If you ever comment on disease management, do it in a positive, neutral way, such as remarking that keeping the medical condition—whether it is asthma, diabetes, epilepsy or something else—stable and under good control will free him to pursue myriad interests and possibilities.

ENCOURAGE YOUR TEENAGER TO BUILD LIFE AS A WHOLE PERSON

Help your teen to realize that he is not defined by special medical needs or physical limitations and help him to discover what he *can* rather than cannot do. Make a list together of celebrities or people you know in the community who have chronic diseases or handicaps and who live happy, productive lives. Role models can be vital to young teens who are feeling different.

"I felt horrible about myself because of my epilepsy until Rob became my Big Brother," says Kevin, twelve, the only child of a divorced, single mother. "It's great when I see him doing anything anyone else can. He has a good job and a nice house. He's married. And because he takes his medication, he hasn't had a seizure for eight years and so he can even drive! That makes me want to take my pills, too, so I can get free of seizures and drive, too. It really makes me feel a lot less lonely to have someone to talk to about how I hate having epilepsy and how I get scared I'll have another seizure in class and how it feels to do that. He understands better than anyone."

While not everyone can have a perfectly matched Big Brother, contacting the Epilepsy Society or the American Diabetes Association (see your local white pages) may make it possible for your teen to find a support group or pen pal that will help him feel less alone and different and begin to see the disease or condition as a small part of who he is.

"I don't feel that diabetes is the central focus of my life," says Nancy Anderson, a young adult who has had the disease since the age of ten. "Having a chronic disease means taking extra responsibility. But being responsible is what growing up is all about. Life isn't easy for anyone, but I believe you can do anything if you want to do it enough. Diabetes is only a small part of who I am. Controlling my diabetes frees me to do all the things I love to do!"

By encouraging your teen to take responsibility for her life and expand her horizons, you will help her improve her self-image. By encouraging her to develop a self-image as a person with a special medical need that is only a part of who she is, you will help her to combat depression and develop confidence and a more positive body image.

The mind-body link, after all, can work in positive as well as negative ways. Teenagers at ease with their bodies and their special physical strengths, weaknesses, needs and abilities will tend to have more hope for building a happy, productive life—now and in the future.

Part VI

TEENAGERS, SEXUALITY
AND DEPRESSION

17

Facts About Teenagers and Sexual Activity

Society in general tends to be ambivalent about teenage sexuality. On the one hand, it is obsessed with and exploits teenage sexuality—through the media, advertising, music and music videos, TV and films—while mandating adolescent abstinence on the other. We bombard our teens with sexual images. For example, in a study of television-show content, Dr. Victor Strasburger, associate professor of pediatrics and director of adolescent medicine at the University of New Mexico School of Medicine, concluded that young people see and hear 15,000 references to sex on TV every year and fewer than 150 of these have to do with birth control or abstinence.

As parents, however, we're frightened for our adolescent children—and with good reason. Sexual activity has never been riskier or more prevalent.

- Recent findings from the Alan Guttmacher Institute in New York: 53 percent of fifteen- to nineteen-year-old girls and 60 percent of boys in the same age range have had sex.
- Teenagers are being identified as the next large risk group for AIDS. In 1993 the National Commission on AIDS warned of the epidemic "threatening a new generation of Americans."
- At the 2005 National HIV Conference, Dr. Lisa Fitzpatrick, an epidemiologist from the Centers for Disease Control, reported that teen girls in the Southern U.S. are being infected with HIV at much higher rates than teens elsewhere in the U.S. Girls thirteen to nineteen represent

eight percent of the new HIV infections in the South, compared with two percent in the rest of the country.

• Condom use among sexually active teens is less than 50 percent, according to figures from the Centers for Disease Control. The exception: 57 percent of teens under the age of fifteen who are having sex are using condoms.

• Two and a half million teens are infected with a sexually transmitted disease each year.

• More than one million babies are born to teenage mothers each year.

• Teens who know or suspect that they might be gay or lesbian are three times more likely than other teenagers to commit suicide.

• Even teens who are not having intercourse may be engaging in risky sexual behavior.

It is no longer enough—if indeed it ever *was* enough—to tell our teens, "Just say no." In order to intervene in ways that are truly helpful we need to understand why teens are having sex, how self-esteem and depression can impact on adolescent sexual choices and how sexuality can be a factor in depression.

Why Are So Many Teenagers Sexually Active?

The following are only a few of the more common reasons cited by sex educators and experts in adolescent health and behavior.

TEENAGERS ARE REACHING PHYSICAL MATURITY AT EARLIER AGES

Teenagers are reaching puberty earlier, with an accompanying surge in sexual feelings, in a society that glorifies sex. A hundred years ago, the average girl didn't menstruate until she was sixteen or seventeen, and she tended to marry soon thereafter. Today the average of menarche is twelve to thirteen.

So the gap between physical maturity and emotional and social maturity has widened. Teenagers today have longer to wait between the attainment of sexual maturity and becoming true adults emotionally, socially and economically. Many teenagers have the physical ability to have sex, and the media (and their friends) encourage them to do so before their emotional growth catches up and enables them to make wise choices about their sexuality.

FAMILY LIFE HAS CHANGED DRASTICALLY

The decreasing amount of intimacy and nurturing in many families causes teenagers to look elsewhere for such comfort and closeness. (Quite often they seek this in sexual activity as the ultimate step toward intimacy.) Many families today lead busy lives with little time for one another and for shared activities and confidences. Financial pressures can tear families apart emotionally. And seeing that adult commitments, either to a marriage or to a career, quite often don't work out, many teens wonder about the value of waiting and deferring pleasure for future possibilities and make the decision to enjoy themselves in the here and now.

Demographers John F. Kanter and Melvin Zelnik of Johns Hopkins University conducted a study of sexually active adolescents and found that among white teenage girls under the age of sixteen, those who had lost a father through death or divorce were 60 percent more likely to have had sexual intercourse than those living in two-parent homes. And the sexually active teens who did come from two-parent families reported that their families were not close and that they were not able to communicate with their parents. For those over sixteen, family closeness did not loom as such a major factor.

Also because of family changes—with more two-career parents or single parents who work outside the home—teens have more privacy and opportunity to have sex in the afternoon before their parents get home from work. "This is prime time for teenage sex," says Dr. Charles Wibbelsman. "A generation ago teenagers were having sex in the backseats of cars. Today teens are most likely to have sex in their own homes while their parents are away, usually at work."

PEER PRESSURE TO HAVE SEX IS STRONG

Despite the considerable risks and despite the flip side of the statistics show-ing that close to half of all American teenagers are not yet sexually active, the teenager who is still a virgin may feel like the last and only one in his school. In addition to actual sexual activity, there is a lot of bragging, exag-gerating and lying about sexual experience these days.

"A lot of us aren't having sex, but we lie and say we are because we don't want our friends to laugh at us," confesses seventeen-year-old Marcus, a se-nior at an inner-city school in Chicago.

For sixteen-year-old Jill, a junior at an affluent Chicago-area suburban school, sexual activity—rather than lying—seemed to be the answer to peer pressure. "I felt sure I was the only virgin left in my crowd," she says. "It got to the point where I just wanted to get it over with and be able to say, like everyone else, that I had done it. I wasn't thrilled by the experience. I kept thinking, 'So what's the big deal?' But I did it because I wanted to fit in and be like my friends."

Those teens who have not yet discovered their own value as human be-ings are especially vulnerable to peer pressure to be sexually active. Those who have plans for the future and who feel good about themselves, on the other hand, are less likely to see sexual acting out as the route to self-fulfillment and acceptance.

"Many teens who become sexually active at a young age have no dreams for the future," says Dr. Paula Duke-Duncan, coordinator of health services for the Burlington, Vermont, school district and assistant clinical professor of pediatrics at the University of Vermont School of Medicine. "They feel they have nothing to lose by engaging in sex—or even having a baby—at an early age."

SEXUAL ACTIVITY CAN BE A FORM OF REBELLION

If parents voice strict prohibitions against sexual activity of any kind and are very controlling in all areas of a teenager's life, he may see sexual acting out as a way to accomplish two goals. First, it is a means of rebelling against parental values, dictates and mores. Second, it is a way of proclaiming separateness, a way of saying "I own my body and I can do whatever I want with it and you don't really have anything to say about it!"

SEXUAL ACTING OUT CAN BE AN ATTEMPTED ANTIDOTE TO OR EXPRESSION OF DEPRESSION

Some teenagers take sexual risks as a way of expressing their depression and low self-esteem. Having unsafe sex has been called "indirect self-destructive behavior" and is particularly shocking when it occurs in circumstances that put young people in very direct danger of infections with the HIV (AIDS) virus.

Two horrifying but not unusual examples of this behavior:

• In April 1993, Planned Parenthood counselors in San Antonio reported that they had seen five teenage girls, aged fourteen and fifteen, who came in for HIV tests after having had sex with male members of a local teen gang who had tested positive for the AIDS virus. The girls bragged to counselors of their "bravery" in engaging in this risky sex as part of a gang initiation practice and said that they were dared to have sex with someone who was HIV-positive.

• Adolescent gay males have turned away from safe sex. According to a 1991 San Francisco Department of Public Health study, 43 percent of the seventeen- to nineteen-year-old gay males surveyed had experienced unprotected anal intercourse and 90 percent had engaged in oral sex without using a condom. In this age group, HIV infection has jumped to 14.3 percent, representing an increase that is almost 40 percent higher than among those twenty-three to twenty-five years old. Their reasons for risking their lives ranged from "Nothing bad will happen to me!" to "Do I want to be around when all my friends are dead?"

For other depressed teens, sex can be an attempted antidote to depression. The depressed teen may hunger for love and attention, acceptance and caring. She may try to find this in sexual involvements. Some teens hope that through sex they will become more loved and valued. They fantasize about sex filling gaps in their self-esteem and making them wise and adult. They dream that sex is the key to true intimacy and commitment.

Having sex for these reasons usually creates even more problems for the teenager because, of course, it does not often meet these high expectations. It does not make one instantly wise and adult, bring acceptance, foster intimacy or guarantee deep and lasting love. It is not even fun and doesn't feel good to some teens whose attempts at sexual sharing may be handicapped by lack of privacy, time, emotional maturity and experience.

While you can't prescribe and mandate what your child's sex life will be like, you *can* have a major influence in this area if you approach the subject of sexuality in an open, firm and caring way with your child.

Sexuality-related problems are particularly distressing to both parent and teenager, but these problems present opportunities for you to educate, communicate with and show your love and commitment to your child. You the parent are crucially important in helping your teenager get beyond this troubled passage, to grow in self-acceptance, responsibility and the capacity to love. This can't be taught in sex education classes, at the movies or in books. It can be taught by you—by what you say, what you do, how you live and how you share feelings and ideas with your teenager. You may not be able to make choices for your teenager. You may not agree with some of the choices he or she makes. But you *can* make a real difference in the way he or she feels and how he or she grows in the capacity for sharing love and joy and intimacy with others.

CHAPTER

18

Crisis Prevention: Raising a Sexually Responsible Teenager

Sexuality is part of all our lives, whatever our choices of expression. All people, from infants to the elderly, are sexual beings and are capable of responding to any number of sensual feelings. Feeling good about one's sexuality is an important part of self-acceptance and the development of strong self-esteem. This, in turn, is a major factor in making responsible sexual choices. It's important to accept one's feelings, whatever these may be, without labeling them as bad or dirty. However, we *are* responsible for *actions*. With these actions come certain moral responsibilities to ourselves and to others. Acting in a caring, responsible way enhances self-esteem, improves relationships and helps to prevent sexuality-related crises.

How can you help your child not deny sexuality or abuse it, but grow into a loving, responsible sexual person?

Take Responsibility for the Sex Education of Your Child

Schools can't and shouldn't do it all. Information from peers is often crude and inaccurate. And information from sex education books, while often accurate and helpful, is purposely general and objective in order to reach a large cross section of people. If you have good communication with your teenager, only you know exactly what he really wants and needs to know.

Only you can discuss sexual choices in the context of your child's own up-bringing and life experience. Since teenagers are bombarded with sex via the media as well as pressure from peers, it's up to you to help your teen make sense of all this and decide which choices are right for him or her.

It isn't an easy position to be in and many parents meet the challenge with confusion or embarrassed silences. A study of 1,400 parents of children twelve and under in the Cleveland area revealed that 88 percent had never discussed sex with their children. Among parents of nine- to eleven-year-old girls, 40 percent had not yet explained menstruation—an alarming number, since today many girls begin menstruating at ten or eleven.

Many parents who grew up in times when sex was not discussed openly find it difficult to change that pattern. Others are afraid that too much talking and too much information will put ideas into their kids' heads. Actually, the more information young people have, the better. A recent study of college students revealed that students who had the most accurate knowledge about sex (measured via a written exam) were less likely to be sexually active. Those who knew the least, on the other hand, tended to be the most sexually active. It is usually what teenagers *don't* know about sex—or what they as-sume to be true—that can hurt them.

Since silence and embarrassment about sex on your part teaches your child more than you realize, it makes sense to take the risk of communicating with and educating your child in a more positive way. Examine your own feelings about sex, with an accent on the positive feelings you have. When you consider your negative views and your embarrassment about the subject, ask yourself where and how you got these attitudes and whether or not you really want to pass them on to yet another generation. Perhaps now is the time to break the chain of embarrassed and awkward silences.

Offering your teenager factual books about sex is a good beginning, es-pecially if you review and discuss the information together. However, if it isn't used in this way—to facilitate communication and to provide solid facts for discussion—a book's ability to help is limited. A book cannot speak to your child in the personal way you can. And "plumbing information"—straight facts about sex—is only part of what good sex education is all about. Your child also needs to know what sexually responsible behavior is, how to make choices that are right and how to grapple with mixed feelings and moral dilemmas.

Explore Ideas and Issues in a Nonthreatening Way

Instead of maintaining silence on the subject of sexuality or defensively asking "Why do you want to know *that*?" when your teenager requests factual information, it is more helpful to give whatever information is requested, finding the answer together if you're not sure of the facts yourself, and to keep moral discussions on a nonthreatening level.

You can do this in everyday situations using a book you are reading, a TV show or movie or the crisis situation of someone you know as the springboard for an informal discussion. Instead of interrogating your teen about behavior, ask for and listen to his or her opinions and perceptions while being open about your own.

A book about sexuality can open a conversation: "I've been reading this book and just discovered something interesting that I never realized before. . . ." or "I was reading this book and I don't know about this part. I'm not sure I agree with it. What do you think?" Or, if a family you know is experiencing a sexuality-related crisis, it may help to explore in a general way how such a crisis happened and how it might have been prevented. Discussing the general issues of premature parenthood in a realistic way can be helpful, for example, since many teenagers romanticize parenthood.

"My daughter was feeling a little envious of a classmate who was expecting a baby because she was getting a lot of attention and was anticipating having a cute, cuddly baby to love," says Carolyn Mager, the mother of two teenagers. "One evening I asked how Cece was doing and remarked that I feared Cece would be in for a shock once the baby came. I shared some of my own feelings about parenthood when I first became a mother at twenty-six: the moments of love and of desperation, the unrelenting demands as well as the joys of children, saying I was glad I was more mature and had had a lot of life experience before I took on the challenge of parenthood. I asked my daughter Lisa how she would feel if she were in Cece's place and if she would choose to be a parent at an early age. It started a really good conversation. I purposely didn't put on what Lisa calls my 'teaching voice.' I just shared ideas and listened to hers. We didn't agree on everything, but we did listen to each other and maybe some of what I said made an impression. That's certainly better than it used to be."

Many parents today feel intimidated by the sheer volume of information young people need to know and parents need to discuss—especially when it involves behaviors that generally have not been part of even the most enlightened parent-child discussions about sexuality: topics such as oral or anal sex, for example. However, given the risks of these behaviors and the fact that teens sometimes engage in them instead of vaginal intercourse to avoid pregnancy or loss of technical virginity, they do need to be discussed. Using a book or magazine discussion of the topic as a lead-in can help: "I read this study here that some teens tend to have anal intercourse. . . . Have you heard of that? Do you know what it means? Do you know how dangerous it is?" You can admit that you're uncomfortable talking about it, but concerned about your teen knowing all the risks so he or she won't take any chances.

Try to see sex education as sharing information rather than always giving it. "When my child asked me a question I couldn't answer or something came up about which I knew little, I used to feel threatened," says one father. "Only when I gave myself permission not to know everything could we really start communicating. I began to say, 'I'm not sure about that. Let's find out the answer together.' I find that when we explore sexual information and issues together, we talk quite easily and my children are better able to accept this information without embarrassment or rebellion."

If the issue of your child's sexual activity has come up, take a less judgmental approach that invites introspection and communication.

"It may help to raise a question," says Dr. Marilyn Mehr. "You might ask, 'Can you have sex in this situation and still feel good about yourself?' or 'Is what you're doing or thinking of doing adding to or taking away from your feelings about yourself as a worthwhile person?' "

Instead of expressing strict prohibitions against teenage sex, state your reservations about such activity and very clearly say why you feel this way.

After your opinions, ask your teenager what he or she thinks about this and explore together what personal responsibility, safe sex and emotional readiness for sex might mean.

Sharing information about sexuality as a natural part of life is a much more effective means of education than the one-time-only excruciatingly embarrassing Big-Talk-About-Life. Exchanging bits and pieces of ideas and concepts on a day-to-day basis puts sex where it belongs—as part of life, as part of one's total identity, not as something mysterious, overwhelming, secret and totally forbidden (and possibly more attractive than ever to the curious teen). Growing up with a balanced view of sexuality and how it fits into one's life in general helps a child get a better perspective and begin to make responsible choices.

Help Your Child Build Healthy Self-Esteem

A glance at magazines aimed at teenage girls points to the crucial importance of self-image: Most of these magazines, subtly or not, have material that can savage a young girl's self-esteem. It isn't simply a matter of models displaying impossible thinness and physical perfection. It's a matter of editorial emphasis on the importance of popularity, boys' opinions and physical attributes over intellectual or emotional growth. While many parents get upset when such magazines ran articles that seem to encourage sexual interest or assume sexual activity, articles such as "Are Smart Girls Sexy?" (a poll of teenage boys that ran in *YM* recently with a resounding consensus of "No!") or *Sassy*'s recent "How These Girls Became Geeks" (featuring three girls who "even though they're pretty" have been condemned to geekdom because they're smart and show it by making top grades) may do more harm and make girls more vulnerable to peer pressure than blatantly sexual articles. Discussing your feelings about such articles and underscoring for your daughter how vital it is that she believe in herself, her rights and her future can be a good start in building self-esteem. You can also help to identify major talents and interests she may have and encourage her to develop them.

If your teenager feels good about himself in most areas of life, he will be less susceptible to peer pressure to have sex (or to engage in any other risk-taking behaviors).

WHAT DO TEENAGERS EXPECT AND WANT FROM SEX?

Some teenagers (and older people, too) seek personal validation through sex. Some look for intimacy. Some expect to find warmth and love through sexual sharing. Exploring your teen's sexual expectations together is an opportunity for you to express the idea that when one comes to a relationship with maturity, a strong and positive sense of self and an overflow of love and warmth to give to another (rather than an emotional void to be filled), the chances for true intimacy—whether or not the relationship also involves sex—are much greater. It is also an opportunity to discuss the fact that sense of self and the ability to validate oneself as a worthwhile person (instead of looking for affirmation from others) grows as a person grows emotionally and intellectually and that good relationships happen as the result of many factors, including time, commitment, good communication and sharing.

WHAT IS RESPONSIBLE SEX?

Someone who is sexually responsible has loyalty to his or her own values, sensitivity and consideration for others and a realistic attitude toward sexual activities and possible consequences. This person

- takes the threat of AIDS and other sexually transmitted diseases seriously and is willing to take the responsibility to protect himself or herself and the partner from risks of infection.
- utilizes reliable forms of birth control to guard against an unwanted or badly timed pregnancy.
- chooses to have sex because the time, the person, the feelings and the circumstances are right. He or she does not have sex out of fear of losing the partner or feeling different from peers. The sexually responsible person feels secure enough to be true to his or her own values, to make free choices about expressing sexuality right now. He or she feels as free to

say no as yes. Choosing not to have sex when the person and circumstances are not right, even at the risk of disappointing someone else, can be a positive choice. He or she doesn't feel the need to prove himself via sexual activity.

• does not use sex to exploit another person. This means seeing a partner as a person, not an object to be used. It means not lying about HIV status, sexual history or feelings or intentions. It means putting an emphasis on sharing, not scoring, and on being a friend as well as a lover. A friend respects another's choices, privacy and feelings and will not try to force another to act against his or her own best interests. A friend will not abandon, ridicule or reject another in a crisis. A friend can enjoy the partner as a complete and separate person who has much to share besides sex.

• has sex within the framework of a caring relationship in which partners have realistic expectations about sex and each other and can communicate openly about feelings, fears, expectations and preferences. They are able to be vulnerable and real with each other.

• is willing to take responsibility for his or her actions, not only in preventing the spread of AIDS and other sexually transmitted diseases or preventing an unwanted pregnancy, but also in taking care to be kind, honest, considerate and caring as a partner.

WHAT IS THE DIFFERENCE BETWEEN SEX AND SEXUALITY?

"Sex" is a description of gender and is often used to mean sexual intercourse. "Sexuality" is part of who we are, a fact of life from birth to death. As such, it is not bad or wrong, but simply a part of our lives. Sexuality is feelings and being in addition to acting.

IS SEX THE BEST WAY TO EXPRESS LOVE AND INTIMACY?

Sexual intercourse can be pleasurable in a number of circumstances and is a special joy when shared within the context of a loving, committed relationship.

But it is not necessarily the ultimate proof of love nor is it always necessary for the development and growth of love between two people. It may help if you and your teen could make a list of all the ways people show love for each other.

"There are many ways of sharing love," says noted sex educator Elizabeth Canfield. "Hearing a concert together is sharing love. Taking care of a loved one who is sick is sharing love. Working together on a project you really believe in is a form of making love. Discovering a lovely flower together, having a good conversation, even sharing a disappointment or sorrow is making love. Love and intimacy mean a great variety of shared experiences, both good and bad. That's what real commitment is all about. It can be fun. It can also hurt. It means committing yourself to struggle and to share."

Making your teenager aware of the many ways of sharing love and the challenges and joys of true intimacy is a vital part of his or her sex education.

Don't Be Afraid to Express Your Own Values

It's important for your teenager to know where you stand. After a period of rebellion and testing, by early adulthood children often come to share parental values quite closely. It's important to express your values even if your teen disagrees. Disagreement and seeming indifference do not mean that you haven't been heard.

In a study presented at the 1992 American Psychological Association meeting in Washington, Dr. Melody Graham of Mount Mercy College in Cedar Rapids, Iowa, found that teens' sexual activity is related to parental attitudes and approval. Researchers surveyed 1,380 students from grades seven through twelve, asking questions about sexual activity, birth control and communication with parents about sex. The findings: Adolescents who knew or believed that their parents would disapprove if they had sex and those who looked primarily to their parents for guidance were less likely to engage in intercourse. Dr. Graham concluded that parents need to be open with their children if they disapprove of adolescent and/or premarital sex.

Avoid Either/Or Thinking

Realize that you and your teenager will probably have clashes of values and some differing ideas about sexual behavior and responsibility. When this happens, it does not mean that your child does not respect you and your feelings. It's important to make clear to your child that mutual love and respect are not dependent on conformity to your values or your child's. At the same time, listening to your teenager's feelings and opinions and accepting them does not mean agreeing with or approving of them. It simply keeps communication open. A clash of values now does not mean that it will always be so. While you may never agree totally with your child's personal choices, you may still wield some positive influence. You may or may not be able to prevent your child from having sex before *you* think the person, time and circumstances are right, but you certainly can influence the level of his or her personal responsibility, whatever his sexual choices, by strongly encouraging your adolescent to be responsible, loving and nonexploitive. These qualities are essential to good self-esteem and rewarding relationships—sexual and otherwise.

It is essential not to reject an adolescent on the basis of his or her sexual behavior. Threats or actual rejection reinforce hurtful patterns of behavior. Your teenager, convinced that he or she is not really loved at home, will look for such unconditional love in others, possibly in sexual relationships, and be vulnerable to a great deal of pain, low self-esteem, disappointment and possible exploitation by others. It is far more constructive to let the child know that he or she is loved, even if you don't love a particular behavior.

Be Open to the Idea of Others Helping

Sometimes the whole area of sexuality is too difficult and overwhelming for a teenager and parent to discuss completely. This may be especially true with parents whose own upbringing and value systems do not include open discussions of sexuality or who find it so awkward and embarrassing that they fear doing more harm than good. It can also be true of a single parent raising a child (especially one of the opposite sex) alone and feeling that he or she can't possibly tell the child everything that's necessary. That's when outside sources can help. Books, school sex education classes and help from extended family members, friends, physicians and others are all valuable.

Contrary to the common fear, knowledge about sex does not equal action. It promotes responsibility. Ignorance, on the other hand, leads to experimentation out of curiosity, exploitation, unwanted pregnancies and the spread of sexually transmitted diseases. Remember: More than ever, it's what teens don't know about sex that can hurt them the most.

19

Facing the Reality of Sexual Activity and Depression

Sometimes the depression comes first and the teenager uses sex in an attempt to anesthetize troubling feelings, seek comfort and love, capture parents' attention or act out in rebellion against parental control.

In other instances the teenager has sex in response to peer pressure or his own curiosity and sexual feelings or as a means of proclaiming separateness from parents—and depression follows. This depression may come as a result of a number of feelings: guilt, rejection by a lover, fear of not being normal, disappointment over the experience and parental anger and rejection, real or anticipated. The young adolescent may have many mixed feelings about the experience.

When a woman we'll call Mrs. Gates brought her sixteen-year-old daughter, Ashley, in to see Dr. Charles Wibbelsman recently, she confided to him that she suspected that Ashley was having sex with her longtime boyfriend and didn't seem comfortable sharing this information with her mother. Mrs. Gates wanted to make sure that Ashley knew about and was practicing safe sex and using birth control and asked Dr. Wibbelsman to talk with her daughter and do whatever physical examinations were in order.

Talking privately with Ashley, he confirmed her mother's suspicions and found that she and her boyfriend had not been using condoms or any form of birth control. The two talked about the importance of both, and Ashley agreed to have a pelvic examination and tests and to use birth control pills and condoms faithfully.

When Dr. Wibbelsman began the gynecological exam, Ashley began to cry. Stopping to comfort her, he asked what she was feeling. "I'm thinking that my mom, whom I love so much, knows that I am having sex and that I will never really be her little girl again," the teen sobbed. "It's like a part of me, a part of our relationship, is gone forever and that really hurts. I hope she isn't disappointed in me! I hope she still loves me as much."

Reflecting on the incident, which ended with mother and daughter tearfully embracing and expressing their love for each other in his office, Dr. Wibbelsman observes that such feelings are not unusual. "Teens care very much about what their parents think," he says. "As rebellious as they may seem, they really don't want to hurt or disappoint their parents or risk losing their love. That's why it's so important to be careful with your teenager's feelings—even when you very much disagree with your child's choices. It's important to disagree or to caution them with love. This can help them to be more responsible and self-respecting in future choices they make."

How You Can Help

DON'T ATTACK OR LABEL YOUR TEEN OR TAKE PERSONAL AFFRONT

If you find that your teenager is having sex, there is an understandable stab of fear: fear about AIDS, about other serious sexually transmitted diseases, about a life-limiting pregnancy and no less fear, perhaps, about your child being hurt or being used. There may be anger that may prompt enraged questions or comments such as "How could you do such a thing?" or "How could you do this to me?" There may be guilt that prompts you to ask yourself, with quiet anguish, "I thought I was a good parent. . . . Where did I go wrong?"

Such feelings are common and understandable, but in order to best help your teen make subsequently responsible choices and to maintain good communication, you need to keep from attacking or labeling your teen or exaggerating behavior (for example, calling a sexually active teen "promiscuous" when he or she may be having sex in the context of a caring, committed relationship). Attacks, labels and exaggerations are hurtful and damaging to self-esteem and to your relationship with your teenager. They close doors when, more than ever before, you need to be open, honest and caring with each other.

KEEP YOUR OWN FEELINGS UNDER CONTROL

You may need to blow off steam to a spouse, a close friend or relative or a professional counselor. Try to discharge your angry, frightened and guilty feelings to trusted others and in ways that will not damage your relationship with your teenager. It's important to realize your limitations, that you probably can't stop sexual activity once it has started. However, you can make your opinions and values clear in ways that will make your teenager listen and really hear what you're saying.

COMMUNICATE YOUR CONCERN IN A CARING WAY

Gently express your love and your fear for your teenager if you discover or suspect that she may be having sex: "I love you and I'm upset over this because I'm afraid that something bad will happen to you. AIDS and other bad things do happen to nice people. It's dangerous to assume that it can't happen to you. It can. I want to talk very openly here about what you're doing to protect yourself and make sure you have all the information you need. You may or may not decide to rethink your decision about having sex, but protecting yourself is a must. I feel very strongly about this because I love you so much."

Beyond these concerns, you may also want to ask your sexually active teen, "How does having sex make you feel about yourself and your relationship? Does it add to or take away from your good feelings about yourself?"

If your teenager hasn't told you that he or she is sexually active, but has left clues for you to find, you might say, "I get the feeling that you want me to know. Maybe you want to talk over some of your feelings. I'd certainly be willing to talk. I'm very concerned about you."

When you simply suspect that your teenager may be having sex, it might be helpful to say, "I see that you and _____ are getting very involved with each other and I feel concerned. I would like us to talk about what close in-volvements, including sexual involvements, can mean."

Since you're unlikely to change the fact that your teen is having sex, however much you might wish to do so, it's important to be gentle in your questions and suggestions as you encourage your teen to examine his behavior without feeling the need to be assertive by disagreeing with you and refusing to listen. If you approach the matter from a caring standpoint, your teen may come to the independent conclusion that some of his behavior needs to change.

If the teenager is upset, worried or depressed, but can't pinpoint the exact feelings he has about a sexual experience, it may help if you make some general observations: "Some people are disappointed in sex at first because they had such high expectations. Some people think that sex will increase closeness or commitment, and there are times when that doesn't happen and it's very disappointing. I don't know if that's what's going on with you, but if it is or if you're feeling troubled about what happened, I'm here to listen and try to understand."

If your teenager is sad about the loss of a lover who didn't call again after a sexual encounter, it is more productive to acknowledge the sadness and disappointment: "You seem to be very sad and upset about this. I understand. You trusted this person and felt deeply for him and it can really hurt when he doesn't call or want to be with you."

Stifle the urge to say, "Well, what did you expect? He got what he wanted! You've been used. When will you ever learn?" Instead, show that you understand your teen's feelings, even if you disapprove of her actions. If you show your child that you care and can be trusted with feelings and confidences, you can discuss in a reasonable fashion the ways the teen might modify behavior to feel better about herself and to prevent such unhappy events in the future.

HELP YOUR TEENAGER FEEL BETTER HIMSELF

Tell him that he is a valuable, worthwhile person and in which ways. Express your love, even when you disagree and as you voice concern. Teens who know they are valued as separate persons and who have good self-esteem are not as likely to get involved in hurtful sexual liaisons and are more likely to take care of themselves in all ways. Explore ways that the teenager can improve self-esteem, deal with depression and express love and commitment, sex being only one of many ways that people say "I care." With empathy and open communication, you may help your teen realize that sex is not the best antidote to depression or a cure-all for low self-esteem. Most of all, you can offer your teenager the warmth, love and support he needs and wants so much.

20

Pregnancy

Hopelessness, passivity, hunger for love and attention and a limited view of the future, as well as ignorance about sex and birth control, often form parts of a tragic emotional equation that can equal teenage pregnancy and parenthood.

The latest figures continue to be alarming:

• An estimated three million teenage girls become pregnant every year, according to figures from the 1993 National Health Council's Forum on Health for Women.

• After falling for more than a decade, teen birth rates rose sharply in the second half of the 1980s, according to figures from the National Center for Health Statistics. In 1990, 60 of every 1,000 teenage girls gave birth, up from 50 of every 1,000 in 1986. (In 1970—before abortion was legal—the rate was 68 per 1,000.) While older teens gave birth more often than younger ones, the birth rate among teens under eighteen rose twice as fast.

• Recent research reveals that girls whose parents have divorced, particularly when the girls are in late childhood, are at risk for precocious sexual activity, pregnancy and nonmarital birth. This was true regardless of race or socioeconomic level.

• Approximately 3,000 teenage girls in the United States will get pregnant today.

• One out of every ten girls between the ages of fifteen and nineteen becomes pregnant each year. Of these pregnancies, five out of six are unplanned.

• Half of all teenage pregnancies occur within the first six months after initial intercourse. Twenty percent of teen girls get pregnant the first *month* they have sex.

Depression can be a significant factor in teenage pregnancy, particularly when the pregnancy is at least partially intentional.

"A teenager may become pregnant as a way of feeling important and needed," observes Dr. Marilyn Mehr. "And this is a way of coping with her depression."

Studies tend to support this observation. In one group of unmarried teenagers who were pregnant for the first time, 36 percent revealed that the pregnancy was intentional. Adolescent-behavior experts observe that the adolescent who gets pregnant on purpose is often depressed, has low self-esteem, has no particular dreams or hope for the future and sees no advantage in waiting for parenthood. She may see a baby as the antidote to her loneliness and lack of accomplishments. She may also use the pregnancy to please or keep a boyfriend or to soothe her feelings of grief over the loss of a loved one through death or a parental divorce. Teen boys with low self-esteem may encourage their girlfriends to get pregnant and see such pregnancies as proof of manhood.

Statistics and general facts about teenage pregnancy are alarming enough but are nothing compared to the shock and desperation you may feel if you discover that your teenage son or daughter is involved in such a pregnancy. In the event of such a crisis, how can you best help?

How You Can Help

TAKE A DEEP BREATH AND THINK BEFORE YOU SPEAK

You are shocked, scared, angry, desperate. You feel like lashing out verbally. You may feel like punishing your teenager. Before you do . . . take a deep breath and consider that the pain of telling you about the pregnancy, planned or not, is usually a punishment in itself for the frightened teen who needs your help, love and support now more than ever before. Your first words will long be remembered, so make sure that your response is memorable in a positive way. Concentrate on feelings before exploring action alternatives. If you can manage it, tell your teen that he or she is loved and that you will do everything possible to help in this moment of crisis. Not only will this help the teenager to cope better, it may also greatly improve your relationship for years to come.

Jeannie Collins is a young adult now, but not so long ago she was a scared sixteen-year-old telling her parents that she was pregnant. "I thought my parents would kill me or throw me out, and I was convinced they didn't love me," she says. "It took a crisis like that for me to realize how wrong I was. They were so supportive. I could tell that they were hurt and disappointed, but they were really there for me and let me know that they loved me and would stick by me. I made the decision to have an abortion. It wasn't an easy decision or experience, but Mom and Dad were there for me and that's something I'll never forget."

HELP YOUR TEENAGER EXPLORE ALTERNATIVES IN A REALISTIC WAY

Sometimes this means helping your daughter or your son's girlfriend deal with a lot of peer pressure. The trend among young mothers—about 96 percent of those who choose not to have abortions—is to keep their babies. Classmates and friends can be cruel and judgmental toward their pregnant peers who choose to place their babies for adoption or to have an abortion. However, many of the young women who choose to keep their babies are making a fantasy-based decision that could negatively influence their lives and the lives of their children for years to come.

It's important, then, to explore *all* alternatives thoroughly and to help the teenager realize that no alternative is painless or trouble-free.

Marriage: The teenage couple who choose to marry face a three times greater risk of divorce than couples who are over twenty. They face a number of educational and financial hardships as well as isolation from friends, whose interests and experiences are suddenly so different. With a lot of love, luck, maturity and emotional and financial help from their families, the young parents may have a chance to beat the odds and build a happy family life, but they would be exceptional.

If you and your teen are considering this alternative, it would be wise for the young couple and their extended families to seek premarital counseling with a marriage family therapist.

Adoption: The teenager who relinquishes a baby for adoption may be praised for a very unselfish act—giving up the baby for its own good to a couple who may be much better equipped in many ways to raise the child. There is undeniable pain, however, in putting one's own child up for adoption.

"I felt a mixture of grief and relief when I gave up my baby," says Sandi, seventeen. "I cried and cried. I'll always wonder about him, but I feel like I gave us *both* a chance at life by making the choice I did."

Some pregnant teens today are opting for private adoptions that may be "open"—allowing the birth mother to know and perhaps even keep in touch with the adoptive parents so that she can keep track, if only through letters and photographs, of her child. If you and your teenager are considering this alternative, do take care to check out the screening procedures for prospective parents and the legal aspects of the adoption process. Generally, it can be safer to work through an established agency such as Crittenden Services or BirthRite, where the birth mother can receive special supportive care and counseling before and after making her decision.

Abortion: Abortion is a controversial option, but one chosen by many teenagers. It is estimated that about one in three abortions in the United States today is performed on a teenager.

Most legal abortions, usually performed in the first three months of pregnancy, are quite safe. While teenagers have a 60 percent higher death rate for pregnancy and childbirth than older mothers, they have the lowest abortion mortality rate.

Emotional aftereffects of abortion vary, depending on how the girl feels about her decision and how supportive her family and friends may be. According to a Harvard study, 91 percent of postabortion patients studied felt relieved and at peace with their choice. Other studies have shown that about 25 percent of patients have postabortion depression. Some feel that this is primarily an emotional reaction, while others contend that it may be due in part to hormonal reactions much like those that occur after childbirth and trigger postpartum blues. Some women, however, feel guilty and upset if they have strong beliefs against abortion or feel that they did not make the choice freely. "If a girl feels forced into an abortion by her parents or boyfriend or if she has strong convictions against abortion, she may have emotional problems afterwards," says pastoral counselor Reverend Hugh Anwyl. "Some of these girls may become pregnant again right away to replace the fetus that was lost."

These comments point to the importance of not forcing alternatives on your teenager. Abortion may or may not be the right choice in your situation, but the teenager's pain will be less if she feels that she played an active role in making the decision.

If you and your teenager are considering abortion, Planned Parenthood affiliates across the nation can offer you a wide range of services, from nonjudgmental counseling to abortion services and follow-up birth-control help and information.

Keeping the baby: Having and keeping the baby is an increasingly popular option among teenagers today, despite the obvious challenges. Many, of course, don't anticipate the demands that infants and small children place on parents or the considerable difficulties of finishing school, raising a child, finding a means of support and taking on years of responsibility at a very young age. Many expect that their own parents will raise their babies, then sometimes resent their help. Others begin a lifetime of welfare dependency.

There *are* success stories, such as seventeen-year-old Johanna, who graduated from high school and is a nursing student at a local community college while her mother cares for her baby. "But as soon as I get home from school, the baby is my responsibility," she says. "And once I finish school, I'm on my own with her. I have no free time and no social life, but if I want to raise my daughter and get an education, this is what I have to do."

Most of the teen mothers who, like Johanna, seem to be doing well are willing to work hard, to make drastic changes in lifestyle and have help from their families. If any one of these elements is missing, the prospects for successful coping with early parenthood are not good.

Family counseling is a good idea if your teenager is considering this option. You need to discuss—as a family—what is possible.

A reality check may help. If you have a relative or friend with a newborn or very young baby, you might ask if you could put your teenage daughter totally in charge of the infant for a day (or better still, for a weekend).

Dr. Charles Wibbelsman suggested this idea to a fifteen-year-old pregnant patient recently. She took care of a friend's baby for a weekend and gained new insights into the demands of parenthood. "She came to the conclusion that she wasn't ready for such responsibility and decided to give her baby up for adoption," says Dr. Wibbelsman. "If a girl can learn about what it's really like to care for a baby and what her limitations might be *before* she gives birth, it can be most beneficial to mother and child."

STATE FIRMLY WHAT HELP YOU CAN GIVE AND WHAT YOU CAN'T

While your emotional support is essential to your teen, it is also important that you make the limits of your ability and willingness to help very clear. This will help your teenager to make realistic choices. Don't let her assume that you will help raise her child if this will not be the case. Explore your feelings about how much or how little you would choose to be involved in caring for the baby. Forget for the moment what you feel you *should* do or what you think *others* feel you should do. Consider what is right and acceptable for you—day by day for the next eighteen to twenty years. Express your feelings gently but clearly to your teen. While there may be some rough times, some disagreements and angry words, making wise and firm choices now may preclude even more pain in the future.

CHAPTER

21

Homosexuality

"Mom . . . Dad . . . I'm gay . . ."

The words may come as an emotional bombshell or as a quiet confirmation of feelings you've had about your teenager for some time.

There may be tears. The tears may express your shock and sorrow as you think about the painful road ahead: the difficulty of being gay in a largely heterosexual and still quite homophobic world; the fact that your beloved child may be hated, harassed, humiliated and rejected simply on the basis of sexual orientation; the fact that these are dangerous times in which to be coming of age sexually—whatever one's orientation—because of the risk of AIDS. The tears may also signal relief that these feelings and thoughts are out in the open, that your child feels safe enough, trusts and loves you enough to risk letting you know him or her in a new way, that this major aspect of your child's life is no longer an anguished secret but a confidence shared.

Beyond the tears, thoughts and feelings may race through your head—some expressed, some unexpressed.

You may feel shocked and quick to deny what your child is telling you: "It's just a phase. . . . How could you possibly know? . . . Everyone goes through a time of wondering who they are. . . . Everyone has crushes on a special teacher or coach or a best friend. . . . Don't worry about it. . . . It will pass. . . ."

You may feel guilty: "What did I do to make you this way? Was it because I loved you too much . . . didn't spend enough time with you . . . tried to raise you as a single parent without enough male influence . . . didn't play sports with you enough . . . ?"

You may feel fear: "You can't be gay! I can't bear the thought of you getting exposed to AIDS and dying! I can't bear the thought of you not being married and having children! I want everything for you. . . . I want your life to be wonderful! I'm scared for you if you are gay! I'm afraid you'll be unhappy and lonely. Most of all I'm scared you'll die a horrible death at a young age. . . . No, please . . . you can't be gay!"

You may feel, beyond the fear, guilt, denial and tears, an overwhelming love for your child: "I love you no matter what. . . . I love you enough to try to understand, to accept anything. . . . I've always loved you and I always will. . . ."

On the way to understanding and acceptance, you may feel an urgent need to know if your teen's feeling that he or she is gay or lesbian comes from a new and deep understanding of self or if it is a matter of taking a passing crush too seriously. You may wonder "Why?" and "What now?"

While it is true that it's very common for young people to develop crushes on same-sex teachers or best friends, and physical experimentation between same-sex friends—especially in early adolescence—is also not unusual, many gay and lesbian teens know that there is a difference.

Kerry, a young woman reflecting back on her recent adolescent experiences, recalls that "I always knew that there was something different about me. As I got into adolescence, all of my dreams and sexual fantasies centered on women. I'll never forget when I was about thirteen and was at a slumber party. We were looking through a dictionary trying to find dirty words. Someone found and read a definition of 'lesbian.' It hit me like a bolt of lightning: 'My God, there is a *name* for what I am!' I'll never forget that moment. It was four or five years after that that I finally told my mother. By that time I had no doubts at all."

Kerry's conviction is mirrored by the findings of a recent Minnesota study of teen sexual orientation. This study of 34,706 Minnesota students in grades seven through twelve suggests that awareness of sexual identity evolves through adolescence, with most teenagers knowing their sexual orientation by the time they are seventeen or eighteen. "At age 12, 26% of the adolescents were unsure of their sexual orientation," reported primary researcher Dr. Gary Remafedi, of the Adolescent Health Program at the University of Minnesota, in the April 1993 issue of *Pediatrics*. "Only five percent were still unsure of their sexual orientation by the age of 17."

So chances are that by the time your teen gets to the point of talking with you about his or her sexual orientation, he or she has a quite clear sense of being gay or lesbian.

Why is your teenager gay or lesbian?

In recent years a number of studies have identified a complex mix of genetic, hormonal and environmental factors that may play a major part in determining sexual orientation.

Much of the research has focused on the questions "Are the brains of homosexuals different from those of heterosexuals?" and "Is there a genetic link to homosexuality? Does it run in families?" All of these have come from an even more fundamental question: "Is sexual orientation an innate or a learned behavior?"

Although research into the causes or underlying factors of sexual orientation—both heterosexual and homosexual—is in its infancy, there have been some interesting findings:

• Dr. Simon LeVay, a former Salk Institute researcher who now heads the Institute of Gay and Lesbian Studies in West Hollywood, California, has found brain differences between gay and heterosexual men. Studying the brains during autopsy, he found that a part of the brain within the hypothalamus, which is responsible for sexual and other basic drives, is smaller in gay men and in women than it is in heterosexual men, pointing to a possible fundamental, biological basis for sexual orientation.

• Dr. Laura Allen and Dr. Roger Gorski at the UCLA School of Medicine have found that the area connecting the two sides of the brain—the anterior commissure—is usually larger in females than in males, but that this area is even larger in homosexual males.

• Dr. Richard Pillard, a Boston University psychiatrist, and J. Michael Bailey, a psychologist at Northwestern University, have conducted joint studies of gays and lesbians and their siblings. The findings have been quite consistent: 52 percent of the identical-twin brothers of gay men and 48 percent of the identical-twin sisters of lesbian women were also homosexual; 22 percent of fraternal-twin brothers and sisters or other biological siblings of gay men and 16 percent of the same in lesbian women shared their sexual orientation; 10 percent of the adopted brothers of gay men and 6 percent of the adopted sisters of lesbian women were also gay or lesbian. These findings point out a real possibility that there is a genetic link, since identical twins share the same genetic makeup and fraternal twins and other siblings have some similar genes. Now the researchers are looking at the identical twins who *don't* share sexual orientation to determine what environmental factors might have had an impact.

• Other studies have focused on environmental factors in the womb, with one theory concluding that stress in the mother during pregnancy can cause hormonal disruptions that affect the developing baby's sexual development and, ultimately perhaps, his or her sexual orientation.

Obviously much research remains to be done, but experts are tending more and more to see sexual orientation stemming more from a complex mix of genetic, hormonal and environmental factors. The prevailing thought is that psychological and social factors alone do not cause homosexuality. Sexual orientation is an intrinsic part of a person's identity and being.

You may be puzzled, however, if you know that your teenager has had heterosexual attractions and experiences, yet is now claiming that he or she is gay or lesbian. It may help to know that in the late 1940s Dr. Alfred Kinsey devised the still widely accepted Kinsey Scale of Heterosexuality and Homosexuality that demonstrated that much of the population falls somewhere in between the two extremes. In a scale ranging from 0 to 6, a 0 would be someone who is exclusively heterosexual and who has never had a profound emotional response, attraction or physical experience with someone of the same sex, while a 6 would be someone with a similarly limited scope of response and experience from a homosexual vantage point. A Kinsey Scale 2 would be predominantly heterosexual with some significant homosexual experience or attraction; a 3 would report equal amounts of heterosexual and homosexual attraction; and a 4, while predominantly homosexual, would have had more than incidental heterosexual experience or attraction.

So a person who is predominantly homosexual may be able to function in a heterosexual way, with varying degrees of satisfaction, but that does not change his or her basic sexual orientation.

For example, Kerry, cited earlier, described herself as a 5 on the Kinsey Scale: "I had sex with two boys when I was in high school, just to see what it was like, but it didn't feel right to me."

For Joe, who describes himself as a 4 on the Kinsey Scale, his heterosexual experience included a number of sexual relationships with women and a brief marriage before he came to terms with his gay sexual orientation at the age of thirty. "I would have accepted myself as gay long before that if I hadn't come from such a strongly religious background and such a conservative family and area of the country," he contends. "I'm sure, deep down, I always knew I was gay. Some of my past sexual experiences with women were very pleasurable . . . but not as satisfying and fulfilling as my experiences with men. My sexual orientation is simply a part of the person I am, and to live a life denying it is no life at all."

It is vital to realize the pain, the vulnerability and the courage that it takes to come to terms with a homosexual orientation in a largely heterosexual world and to share who one really is with the people who matter most.

"I have known, in some way, that I'm primarily attracted to women since I was about seven," says Terri, now a young adult. "I accept myself completely. I can talk easily to friends about being lesbian, but it's much harder to come out to your family. If they reject you, it *really* hurts. There's so much more at stake emotionally, so much more to lose. Sometimes I think 'homophobia' should be spelled 'home-ophobia' and defined as fear of coming out at home."

Risk-taking behavior, which can be a component of depression in adolescents, can be a particular danger among gay teenagers—and a major fear for those who love them. Although AIDS and safe sex have been inculcated into the national consciousness over the past two decades, the "It can't happen to me!" mind-set poses a particular problem with some gay adolescents. Substance use and abuse can impair judgment. And if a teenager is significantly depressed, risk-taking can be passively suicidal in nature.

Josh, now 21, had his first gay sexual encounter at 14. Although he remembers his first experience as positive, Josh had a lot of negatives in his life: feeling different because he has epilepsy only partially controlled by medications, rejection from some family members who shunned him because his sexual orientation clashed with their religious beliefs, and conflicts between his divorced parents. During his senior year of high school, he started drinking and using drugs. By then, he was sexually active with older men, some of whom urged him to have sex without condoms.

"I knew very well the importance of safe sex and condom use," he says. "But I wanted to be accepted by my new friends. And my substance abuse caused me to make some pretty poor choices—in partners and behavior. I didn't have many sober moments during my late teens and I took sexual risks that I would never have taken otherwise. I mean, I grew up reading and admiring Paul Monette's books. I grieved his death from AIDS, even visiting his grave several times. I knew how devastating AIDS can be . . . and yet I took risks. Part of me didn't feel that I was worth safeguarding and part of me didn't care because I was drunk. But what this has meant, unfortunately, is that I am twenty-one-years-old and HIV positive. But that doesn't mean I don't have hope or plans for my life. I'm in college. I'm planning a career in psychology. I'm planning a future, but it's a future complicated by HIV."

For other gay teens, the notion of suicide is much more specific. In a review of professional literature regarding risk factors for suicide in gay and bisexual youth, Dr. Gary Remafedi of the University of Minnesota's Adolescent Health Program, and his colleagues Dr. James Farrow and Dr. Robert Deisher at the University of Washington in Seattle, found that in one sample of 5,000 homosexual men and women, 40 percent had seriously considered or attempted suicide. In another study of 1,000 black and white homosexual young adults, the black homosexuals were twelve times more likely than their heterosexual peers to report thoughts of suicide. The white gay males studied had a three times greater likelihood of suicidal ideation.

In their own study of 137 gay or bisexual males between the ages of fourteen and twenty-one, Drs. Remafedi, Farrow and Deisher found that 30 percent of the subjects had made at least one suicide attempt and half of these had made more than one attempt. While one-third of the attempts were related to personal or interpersonal turmoil regarding homosexuality, many more were made in the same year that the young men had identified themselves as bisexual or homosexual.

Other researchers have found similarly alarming results. For example, a study at San Jose State University estimated that some 600,000 California children are gay, lesbian or bisexual and that a third of this group will become chemically dependent and half as many will attempt suicide.

Given this array of facts and feelings, what can you do when your teenager comes to you and tells you that he or she is gay or lesbian?

How You Can Help

KEEP YOUR FEELINGS UNDER CONTROL

There are some terrible things that people say when they're shocked and in pain. Unfortunately, these things are not easily forgotten. Joe's mother, for example, screamed, "I'd rather see you dead than homosexual!" Both Joe and his mother knew that these words were uttered under stress and not from the heart, but, reports Joe, "they hung there between us for a long time, causing some emotional estrangement. We resolved our differences long ago, but the echo of those words still hurts when I remember."

Even more terrible, perhaps, are ultimatums such as "If you're going to be gay, get out! You can't live here anymore!" Such an ultimatum may be, in effect, a death sentence for an adolescent sent out to live on the streets, who may end up supporting himself via prostitution.

If you're feeling too shocked, angry or heartsick to carry on a reasonable conversation, say so and call a time-out. You might say something such as "I really want to listen and to talk about this, but right now I need a little time to sort out my feelings about all this. Can we talk a little later? I love you and I want to talk. I do want you to know that."

This postponement, while certainly not preferable to an open, caring, on-the-spot conversation, is more beneficial than an impassioned showdown.

Keep in mind that as you begin to communicate with your teen about his or her sexual orientation, troubling feelings and fears are likely to come up again and again. That's why it may be helpful to find a group in which you can share and vent these feelings. Parents and Friends of Lesbians and Gays, Inc. (PFLAG) has more than 200 chapters across the United States and additional groups in Canada and six other countries. You can find a chapter nearest you, online support and information and a complete list of resources by going to the PFLAG website at www.pflag.org.

REAFFIRM YOUR LOVE

The unconditional love of a parent is irreplaceable, and its loss is a terrible blow to a young person. In the midst of your shock and confusion, if you are able to express love for your child, it will do a great deal for him or her and for your relationship. It may even prevent tragedy.

Kara Ogilve first realized that she was lesbian when she was only thirteen, and hating the fact that she was different from her peers, she tried to drown her feelings with alcohol, drugs and sex with boys. "By that time I was so depressed that I was on the verge of killing myself," she says. "I really didn't want to live anymore. Then one day my mother came to my room where I was lying on the bed, crying as usual, put her arms around me and told me that she loved me, would always stand by me and would never put me down for being who I was. She had guessed my secret. I can't tell you what a difference it made. I didn't feel alone anymore. Eventually my whole family came to know and accept my feelings, but it was Mom—a really beautiful lady—who reached out to me first and helped me to feel truly loved again."

Expressing love will keep you in touch with your teen and able to help if help is needed. It will also prevent the real tragedy of unnecessary estrangement just when you and your child need to talk and be there for each other the most.

EXPRESS YOUR CONCERNS WITH LOVE

There are definite hazards to being different and being gay. If you find yourself wanting to express these concerns and reservations, let your child know that they're coming from love: "I love you so much and I feel so much fear and pain when I think of . . ."

Then you can explore the possibilities. The fact is that not all gay men are HIV-positive or will get AIDS. Monogamy and safe sex are safeguards that are increasingly popular in both homosexual and heterosexual young adults. It's entirely possible that your child *will* find a lover with whom to share his or her life (as we know, heterosexuality carries no guarantees for happy or lasting relationships), and increasingly, homosexual families are including children—both biological and adopted. It is quite possible that your child, coming from a loving home, will continue to have love in his or her life—and that life may be a very full and satisfying one.

IF YOUR TEEN SEEMS TROUBLED, SUGGEST PROFESSIONAL HELP

If your teen is depressed or otherwise troubled, professional help may be in order. But don't drag your child to a psychiatrist, psychologist or professional counselor-psychotherapist just because he has revealed his homosexuality.

According to guidelines of the American Psychological Association and the American Psychiatric Association, homosexuality is *not* a mental illness or psychological disorder. The focus in therapy these days with homosexual patients is affirmative: helping them to understand and accept who they are instead of trying to change their orientation.

Therapy aimed at changing sexual orientation has largely fallen out of favor among mental-health professionals because it incorrectly assumes that homosexuality is a disorder to be cured, and because in most cases it simply doesn't work. The relatively few mental-health professionals who do practice such therapy tend to have a strong, fundamentalist religious orientation, as do many of their patients. Religious beliefs may form a very motivating reason to change, but the prevailing thought these days is that such therapy may, for a time, change sexual *behavior,* but it does not change one's basic orientation and feelings.

So it's important to approach therapy with flexible expectations, the primary one being that you would like to see your child feel better about himself or herself and live a happy, productive life, whatever his or her sexual orientation happens to be.

Your loving support will help your teenager to grow in self-acceptance and in his or her capacity to give and receive love in an intimate way.

"What matters most is not whether a person is gay or straight, but how he or she manages relationships," says Reverend Robert H. Iles, a pastoral counselor in Pasadena. "The ability to give and receive love and the capacity to have a truly intimate relationship are so important."

Part VII

SUBSTANCE ABUSE AND OTHER RISK-TAKING BEHAVIOR

22

When Your Teenager Has a Problem with Substance Abuse or Other Risk-Taking Behavior

Peter was twelve when he took his first drink from his parents' liquor supply. Now, six years later, that night still stands out in his memory. "That was the night I became an alcoholic." he says. "I remember I took little drinks from all the bottles in my parents' bar while they were out. I figured that they wouldn't notice any missing that way. I got very drunk and very sick and fell into bed before they got home. I don't think they knew for a long time that their model son was a drunk. That was just the beginning. It got so I kept whiskey in my locker at school and rushed to take a drink between every class. I needed it to get through the day. I also needed booze to get through a party or other social occasion because I was sort of shy and didn't like myself much. Drinking always made me feel better, for a while at least. But it eventually got me into lots of trouble at school, lost me some friends, caused countless hassles with my parents and finally got me in trouble with the police. I was arrested for drunk driving last year. That was when I decided to go to Alcoholics Anonymous. Things are better for me now. I've been sober for eleven months, but it's tough. I'm having to learn how to face my feelings and find new ways to cope with situations booze got me through before. I figure that emotionally and socially I'm about thirteen years old, so I have some catching up to do."

The past year has been one of continuing crisis for Elisa Donnelly, who just turned fifteen. Her parents were divorced and her mother remarried as soon as the divorce was final. She doesn't get along with her stepfather. There have been two moves, a change of schools and the loss of her best friend, whose family moved out of the state. Elisa has been coping with her depression by running away from home every time it all becomes too much for her. The first time, seven months ago, she stayed overnight with a friend. Two weeks ago, Elisa ran to a special shelter and counseling facility for teens. She's still there, getting counseling and thinking through her options. Her mother is troubled about their future. "We've all had a lot of stress this year," she says. "But now every time anyone disagrees with or tries to discipline Elisa, she takes off or threatens to. This running-away habit is very stressful and manipulative. We're getting counseling, but it's hard to know what to do. I'm scared she'll keep running and running farther and maybe end up getting raped or being forced into prostitution and getting AIDS or something. I'm really scared for her. At the same time, I'm furious with her. Her threats and actions are beginning to ruin my life—all our lives—and it makes me mad as hell!"

Pam Mariano's parents are also frightened and furious since their daughter was caught shoplifting at a local department store. Pam had cash in her purse to pay for the earrings she was lifting, but did it, she says, "just to see if I could get away with it."

"We've always tried to teach her values, and she's never gone without anything she really needed," says Pam's mother. "I can't understand why she took such a stupid risk. It's humiliating, but even more, it's frightening because I don't think even Pam knows exactly why she did it."

Risk-taking behavior—from substance abuse to running away, shoplifting, having accidents or driving recklessly—can in many instances be linked with depression.

"Teenage boys, especially, may express their depression via alcohol use, power and speed," says Dr. Lee Robbins Gardner. "Being accident-prone is also a form of self-destructive behavior. If your teenager has a lot of accidents, he may be upset or depressed. When one is depressed, poor judgment and impulsivity are often present and make accidents more probable."

Dr. Calvin Frederick observes that "risk-taking behaviors—including a continuous pattern of accidents, other self-destructive behavior and substance abuse—are frequently indicative of underlying depression. There is a definite correlation between depression and drug abuse and alcoholism and suicide."

Dan Jones, a youth counselor in New Orleans, says that most of the runaways he has seen are not in search of adventure, but are looking for help for a variety of emotional problems and family crises. "Many come from situations where they have lost a parent by divorce or death," he says. "A number have alcoholic parents, and some are running away from abusive situations. I would say a fair number are quite depressed."

Quite often risk-taking behaviors occur in clusters. For example:

- Adolescents who smoke cigarettes and drink alcohol are more likely to engage in other risk-taking behavior if the onset of such behavior occurs in early adolescence, according to a study of risk clusters by Dr. Charles Irwin and Dr. Susan Millstein at the University of California, San Francisco.
- According to the Centers for Disease Control (CDC), alcohol was a major contributing factor in 42 percent of the fatal automobile accidents among sixteen- to twenty-four-year-olds. The CDC has also linked alcohol to other injuries such as falls, burns and drownings.
- A recent Stanford University study of high school sophomores found that both male and female bulimics—those who engage in binge-purge eating behavior—were at greater risk for abusing alcohol than their classmates.
- In a study of 133 consecutive teenage suicides in San Diego, researchers found that the main psychiatric diagnosis for 53 percent of them was substance abuse. Since many deeply depressed young people turn to drugs or alcohol in a futile attempt to alleviate their pain, this cluster may be easily, if painfully, understood.

These risk-taking behaviors can take a dramatic toll on family life and on the quality of life a teenager has now and in the future. And when depression is a component of the risk-taking behavior, as it often is, the result can be a troublesome, even life-threatening cycle of ever-deepening depression.

"A number of depressed teenagers drink alcohol, which is a depressant," says family therapist Shirley Lackey. "It can become a vicious cycle: The teen is depressed and drinks. He may feel better for a while, but then he feels worse and even more depressed."

Risk-taking behavior is not only a physical threat and a means of perpetuating depression, it also cripples a teenager's ability to cope with troublesome feelings and stress. Alcohol and drug abuse are ways a teenager tries to escape from the growing pains of adolescence, from the pressures of learning to get along in the adult world, from the necessity of establishing a strong and separate identity. So risk-taking behavior can exact a high emotional and social price when the adolescent does not pick up the essential life-coping skills usually learned during this time. The fact that teens may attempt to escape problems rather than face them and grow as a result is not surprising to many therapists.

"Substance abuse, which is a very common acting-out behavior for depressed teenagers, is actually taught to our kids," contends Dr. Marilyn Mehr. "Drinking alcohol and use of prescription drugs such as tranquilizers are widespread habits among adults. Kids have a model in us. They get the message: 'If you feel bad, take something.' So they take something instead of *doing* something constructive and learning to cope with their feelings."

Parents can play a major role in helping their teenager to overcome risk-taking habits by identifying problem areas, serving as good role models and encouraging their teens to get expert help in a crisis. Being alert to signs of substance abuse and knowing how to act in risk-taking crises are important steps in improving not only your teen's present life, but also his or her prospects for the future.

23

Substance Abuse

Maybe the alarm bells went off in your head the second time your child came home from a party drunk. Or maybe it's the change of personality—the withdrawal, fatigue, lying and secretiveness—that gave you the feeling that something was wrong. Maybe it's the fact that her eyes are red, dull or blood-shot and that she is suddenly using eyedrops with alarming regularity, claiming it's all just an allergy. Or maybe the changes have been subtle: a new and different kind of best friend, more frequent colds, loss of interest in hobbies. As the symptoms and signs add up, you may begin to wonder if your child has a problem with substance abuse.

Who is most likely to develop a substance-abuse problem?

• *Teens who are depressed:* In several studies, researchers have found that depressed teens are at particularly high risk for drug abuse. Other studies, which included alcoholics and cocaine users, have found that when patients are given treatment for depression and anxiety disorder, alcohol and drug intake diminish as well, indicating that clinical depression may precede and be a factor in causing substance abuse.

• *Teens who have a substance-abusing parent:* According to statistics from the National Council on Alcoholism, children of alcoholics have four times the risk of developing an addiction to alcohol than do children of nonalcoholics. Experts feel that in addition to the power of the role model, there may be a genetic predisposition to substance abuse.

• *Teens who believe that alcohol or drugs will have a positive impact on their lives:* A study at the University of South Florida in Tampa found that young teens at highest risk for substance abuse believed that alcohol would help them to perform better socially, be more popular, be better coordinated and even to think better.

• *Teens whose friends use and abuse substances:* Peer pressure can be overwhelming, especially for the teen with low self-esteem. Of this group, those most at risk for continuing to use and developing lifetime problems with substances are those who use drugs or alcohol to dull pain or find pleasure.

Overall, illicit drug use has declined among teenagers today. In a poll of high school seniors, the National Drug Institute found that the use of illicit drugs had dropped from a high of 54 percent of high school seniors to a low of 33 percent in 1990, and the rate is still falling with use of such drugs as marijuana, cocaine, crack and PCP on the decline.

However, alcohol use is still very high among teens. According to a 1991 survey by the U.S. Department of Health and Human Services, some eight million teenagers, or more than one-third of high school students, drink alcohol weekly, and nearly half a million are "binge" drinkers who consume an average of fifteen drinks a week.

And there are other dangers right in your own home: Teens today are abusing prescription drugs and inhaling household substances with sometimes fatal results. The latter habit, called "huffing," is a growing practice among young teens who inhale household solvents, glue, typewriter correction fluid and the like. The fumes affect the central nervous system and can cause paralysis, cardiac arrhythmia and sudden death in a tragically random fashion.

Another special danger for teens today: use and abuse of anabolic-androgenic steroids. These are synthetic derivatives of testosterone, the male sex hormone, and are used by some athletes to build muscle mass and strength quickly. Use of these dangerous drugs has trickled down to high school athletes and bodybuilders. These drugs can trigger aggressive, violent behavior and lead to a variety of physical problems, including liver damage, high blood pressure, a decreased level of male reproductive hormones and permanent short stature, and some researchers suspect that there may be a link between these steroids and certain forms of cancer.

What Are the Signs of Substance Abuse?

- Sudden rage reactions and aggressive behavior. If these traits occur in an athlete or a teen who has experienced a fairly recent or sudden transformation in muscle mass, this may be a sign of anabolic-steroid use.
- Fatigue, stupor, slurred speech.
- Physical evidence in the trash: a lot of Scotchgard or spot-cleaning canisters, liquor bottles or beer cans. Be alert, too, for prescription drugs or alcohol missing from your own supply.
- A pattern of drunkenness, partying, missing school because of hangovers and/or a variety of physical ailments.
- A formerly fastidious teen neglecting his or her appearance.
- A sudden inability to concentrate.
- Red eyes and the frequent use of eyedrops.
- Memory blackouts.
- Lost time from school due to drinking or drug use.
- Drug paraphernalia such as pipes, cigarette rolling materials, a water pipe or bong, roach clips or bags of unidentified substances (that your teen claims to be "keeping for a friend").
- Irregular eating habits and loss of weight combined with occasional cravings for sweets.
- A hostile, secretive attitude.
- Money or other valuables missing from your home.

If any of these look familiar, this is a good time to keep a close watch on your child. If more than a few look familiar, take action immediately to help your child.

How You Can Help

CONFRONT YOUR TEENAGER WITH YOUR SUSPICIONS

Some parents avoid confrontations because they are afraid of creating more distance between themselves and their children. Others simply don't know what to do. But parental noninvolvement is often interpreted as not caring, so having the courage and commitment to confront your teenager in a caring way is important.

"When you see your teenager in real trouble, you really do need to confront him," says Dr. Marilyn Mehr. "Make your expectations clear and offer to help in any way you can. It's vital to express yourself clearly. You might say, for example, 'I believe that you're an alcoholic and that you need help.'"

Your teenager may be less than thrilled with your observation and may act angry or resentful or may deny that drugs are a problem. Denial is a frequent reaction to such a confrontation. Never try to confront your teenager while he or she is under the influence. Instead, choose a time when he or she is feeling a little down or sick as the result of the habit, or at least when he or she is sober enough to hear what you are saying.

ASSESS YOUR TEEN'S SITUATION

If your teen's pattern of substance use is mild and occasional, this is a time to look at underlying factors and stresses that may be contributing to his or her behavior. Has there been a family move or illness or divorce? He may need some counseling to deal with feelings around these issues or some encouragement from you that he is loved and valued and that things will get better with time.

If your teen has a more than occasional substance-abuse pattern and is beyond responding to your rules and confrontations—for example, if he ignores you and just takes off whenever he feels like it—professional help is in order. This may be individual counseling, especially if the substance-abuse problem has grown from depression, stress and other identifiable factors. If he or she has a persistent, pervasive substance-abuse problem, inpatient treatment in a residential drug- or alcohol-treatment program and/or involvement with a Twelve-Step Program such as Alcoholics Anonymous (many chapters have special groups for teens) may be in order.

Discuss the matter with your teen's physician or with a school principal or counselor or a professional psychotherapist to sort out your alternatives and get the right kind of help for your teen as quickly as possible.

SET FIRM RULES AND GUIDELINES

You will have to set down very firm guidelines, especially if your teenager is not receptive to reasonable discussion and self-examination. Some rules to spell out include:

- No drugs or drug use in the house.
- A strict curfew.
- Modified grounding for repeat offenses, allowing the teen to leave home only to go to school or to sources of help such as counseling.
- No use of the family car until the substance-abuse problem is under control.
- No parties or gatherings at your home, especially when you are out.
- No unexplained phone calls or secretive comings and goings.

You may not win any popularity contests, but you may get a handle on the situation and eventually earn your teenager's respect. You must be willing to say, "This is my house. I make the rules and this is what I will not tolerate."

CUT OFF YOUR TEEN'S CASH FLOW

This means careful monitoring of his allowance and keeping close tabs on goods that could be pawned or sold. You may want to keep expensive jewelry, collector's items, heirlooms, silver, gold and other possessions of value under lock and key, in safekeeping with a trusted friend or relative or in a safe-deposit box.

MAKE IT UNCOMFORTABLE FOR YOUR TEENAGER TO CONTINUE THE HABIT

Don't rush to rescue him every time he gets into trouble as the result of his substance abuse. If you protect him from the consequences of substance abuse, you help to perpetuate the habit.

"When Eric's teachers complained that he was sleepy and inattentive in class, I defended him and suggested that maybe something was the matter with the classes," says Gwen, the widowed mother of sixteen-year-old Eric, who recently completed treatment for alcohol and marijuana addiction at a local facility. "When he was arrested for drunk driving, I was right there to bail him out of jail, even though I was very upset with him. In retrospect, I should have listened to the teachers and let him spend a night in jail."

Letting your teenager face a confrontation with school authorities over unauthorized absences caused by substance abuse (instead of writing excuses for him or her) or even allowing your teen to spend a night in jail may be necessary steps toward the teen's realization that substance abuse is a problem, not an answer.

"If your child has an alcohol or drug problem, see how these substances are taking care of your child's needs and pain," says Dr. Alan Berman. "If the substances are working well, he may reject your help and think you're out of your mind to suggest other sources of help and gratification. But if he is experiencing secondary problems as a result of the habit, he will be more receptive to your suggestions."

FIND AND USE YOUR BEST SOURCES OF HELP

It is quite likely that you alone will not be able to help your teenager overcome a substance-abuse problem, so it's important to realize your limitations both to change your child and to reach him in this crisis.

"You may not be able to help your addicted teenager anymore," says Dr. Mehr. "You can't *make* someone stop drinking or taking drugs. The individual must make this decision and take this step himself."

There are many sources of help worth exploring. Your family physician or psychotherapist may be able to refer you to some of these, which would include treatment centers, groups such as Alcoholics Anonymous, Al-Anon (for families of alcoholics), parental support groups and your local Family Service organization.

By insisting, even forcing, your addicted teen to get help, you may need to "love him enough to let him hate you." That became the motto of comedienne Carol Burnett and the late Joe Hamilton when their daughter Carrie was addicted to drugs during her teen years. Calling their daughter "a walking chemical" during that period and realizing that she had no motivation to help herself, the Hamiltons forced her to go to a drug-treatment program and she eventually recovered. In a number of interviews since that time, Ms. Burnett has stated that parents may need to force their addicted teenagers to get help. "Don't be afraid of your children," she has said. "Don't be afraid they will hate you. Love them enough to let them hate you."

Overcoming a substance-abuse problem may take not only expert professional help, but also time. Some backsliding is common. There are no easy solutions, but there is hope—if you have the courage and the commitment to face your child's substance-abuse problem and reach out for help.

24

Running Away

A very young Judy Garland, her voice tremulous and wistful, closes her eyes and repeats over and over: "There's no place like home. . . . There's no place like home. . . ."

Watching this holiday presentation of *The Wizard of Oz* in the TV room of a youth runaway shelter in St. Louis, fourteen-year-old Wendy stares at the screen with vacant blue eyes. If this were a neatly scripted Hollywood scene, Wendy would nod with recognition, eyes suddenly full of hope. But this is real life and it's painful and not so neatly resolved. Her eyes stay vacant as she turns down the television and tells her story.

"My parents always drank a lot and then they got divorced three years ago and right away they married other people," she says, nearly whispering, wrapping a blanket tightly around her in a comforting cocoon. "The other people didn't want to bother with a kid. It caused problems. Nobody wanted me. I could tell. I'd get upset and cry and fuss and feel like killing myself. My dad doesn't want me for sure, and I felt like I had to run away to save my mom's marriage. She hasn't asked me to come back so I know . . . I know . . ."

Wendy rests her head on her knees, rocking gently, as she recounts the terror of her three days on the streets: days of being cold, scared and hungry . . . and, on the second night out, she was viciously assaulted by a man who dragged her into an alleyway and tried to rape and then strangle her. Brushing her long, blond hair aside, she matter-of-factly points out the purplish bruises and cuts on her neck, then snuggles farther into her blanket. "I'm scared because I don't know what's going to happen to me," she says. Her eyes are suddenly bright with tears. "I need a lot of help and caring right now. . . ."

Sixteen-year-old Kevin is polite, clean and a little shy as he checks in at the West Hollywood Youth Clinic complaining of an ear infection. He is slight and slim and looks even younger than his tender years. After a few minutes it's obvious that this is a bright, well-educated boy. How could he be living on the streets?

Slowly his story emerges. The only son of a rich and powerful corporate CEO, Kevin grew up in an affluent suburb of Los Angeles enjoying the best of everything: private schools, music lessons, vacations abroad. Then his father discovered a letter Kevin had received from a male friend in Switzerland, a friend who had, the previous summer, become Kevin's lover.

There was little discussion about Kevin's gay feelings or lifestyle. His father confronted him. Kevin answered truthfully. His father threw him out of the house that night and he was now living in a Hollywood gay youth shelter and working as a busboy in a trendy restaurant. He tries hard not to cry as he describes his new life: "I'm scared," he says. "I wrote to my friend in Switzerland and told him he could get in touch with me at the restaurant. I hope he sends me a ticket. I don't know what to do . . . just keep healthy and keep hoping, I guess. What else can I do?"

Wendy and Kevin represent a large portion of today's runaway teens. They're neither adventurers nor rebellious adolescents, but teens tested and troubled by life's circumstances. Some, like Kevin and Wendy, are virtual throwaways. Of the 1.2 million teen runaways in the United States each year, an estimated 300,000 have little hope or chance of returning home. They have run from abuse or rejection or chaotic family lives that have no room for them.

But not all situations are as hopeless. Jane, sixteen, is Wendy's roommate at the runaway shelter and is an excellent student and aspiring journalist whose bout of clinical depression and subsequent problems with substance abuse caused her to run away from her comfortable Chicago home. "I thought my parents didn't care," she says. "We couldn't communicate. All that seemed to matter were my grades and the honors I won. They didn't see me as a person. It really hurt. It did. I started drinking and taking pills. They didn't say anything. I got really scared and felt like I had to get away. So I got on this bus as far as my money would take me. . . ."

Whether the causes are severe family problems or more subtle misunderstandings and dysfunctions, runaway behavior is usually a symptom of many underlying family problems. This risk-taking behavior is the culmination of other crises.

How You Can Help

NEVER USE THROWING A TEEN OUT OF THE HOUSE AS A THREAT OR A DISCIPLINARY MEASURE

Many parents try to get tough right away and end up regretting the move. Instead, use all available crisis-management strategies, including professional counseling.

If your conflict is a present or potential stepfamily crisis, keep in mind that most blended families go through a rough period of adjustment that can last as long as two to three years. If your family is having trouble and you're not able to resolve it, family therapy or pastoral counseling can help to smooth the adjustment.

Whether your teen has school problems or substance-abuse problems, has told you he is gay or is almost unbearably moody, face the problems together—with help.

To be fair, many parents are exhausted and exasperated and they don't realize the terrible dangers of life on the streets. Be an informed parent and examine every possible alternative.

REGARD RUNAWAY THREATS (OR SHORT RUNAWAY EPISODES) AS A CRY FOR HELP

Don't dismiss threats or episodes as manipulative or bad behavior. Instead of saying, "So go!" try saying, "I'm concerned and want to know why you feel like running away."

If your teen says things are hopeless, that you'll never understand, offer some hope: "I know it looks that way to you. It's hard for all of us. But let's face this and talk about it. Together we might come up with a solution."

It may help to point out that running away can only postpone solutions and complicate a teen's problems, sometimes tragically.

If your teen has run away to a friend's house for a night or two, this is a vital early warning sign. Start talking with each other. Seek professional help before the runaway behavior becomes more serious and risky.

BE OPEN TO CRISIS HELP AND INTERVENTION

There *are* alternatives to a "shape up or ship out!" ultimatum. There *are* alternatives to the frustrating cycle of anger and desperation in your family. There are times when problems can't be solved by and within the family, when outside professional help can be a relief to all concerned.

IF YOU NEED TIME APART, KEEP IT POSITIVE AND SAFE

There are times when parents and teens need a vacation from each other. This can be accomplished in ways that protect the teen from harm and the family from irreconcilable division. Maybe the teen with benefit greatly by spending a summer with grandparents or with other trusted relatives or friends. Maybe an occasional weekend away with a favorite relative or a friend will give some relief from family conflict. Often one or both parents can benefit from a time-out, too. Taking time out from each other can be a way to clear the air and find new resources and energy to cope.

WELCOME YOUR TEEN HOME

If your teen has run away and then calls asking to come home or appears at the door, this is not a time to vent your anger or punish him or her by denying permission to come back. Welcome him back and then make an effort together to work out whatever problems came between you. This will not only help to heal the rift between you, it is also a step toward resolving troubled feelings. Your open arms and open heart could, quite literally, save your teen's life.

25

Other Risk-Taking Behavior

Shortly after his older brother died of leukemia, Mark Salant, seventeen, began drag racing whenever he could get the family car for a night. In the course of his adventures, he has received two speeding tickets and has been involved in a moderately serious accident that did expensive damage to the car and put Mark in the hospital overnight with a broken arm, cuts and bruises.

Pam Mariano's adventures in shoplifting, on the other hand, have no clear-cut reason or starting point. She has always been something of a loner, shy and retiring with few friends, and she looks considerably younger than her fifteen years. Although her mother noticed expensive clothing in Pam's closet several times before, her shoplifting did not become a family issue and a crisis until she was caught recently by a department-store detective.

It is quite possible that both Mark and Pam engaged in various risk-taking behaviors in response to underlying depression. Shoplifting, reckless driving, vandalism and accidents occur as the result of many factors, of course, including peer pressure, alcohol or drug use or rebellion. But these acts can also be linked with depression.

Some mental-health professionals believe that in many instances shoplifting is associated with depression and shoplifters take things to comfort and reward themselves. Because they feel essentially deprived (of love or material comforts), they believe that they deserve to have what they steal. Others contend that the shoplifter has poor self-esteem and an underlying desire to be caught and punished.

Studies at Baylor University and the University of Colorado have linked rash, impetuous behavior with depression. Such behavior may occur in conjunction with a series of "accidents" that are thinly disguised suicidal behavior.

"I remember a student who was identified by school authorities as a possible suicide because of his obvious depression and his many accidents," says Mary Ann Dan. "He got some supportive therapy and special classes, but is now back in regular classes and is active in football and competitive biking. He's doing well academically, but I still worry about him. He is still having a lot of accidents: several bike crashes in the last few months—more than one would normally have even in competitive situations. This continuing pattern of accidents may indicate that he is still feeling suicidal."

Looking at her current roster of students who require home tutoring, Ms. Dan notes that half of these were injured in single-car crashes. "And all but one or two of these were marginal students with a variety of problems in their lives," she says. "Their accidents could well be indicative of suicidal feelings."

How You Can Help

BE PREVENTION-MINDED

If your teenager is troubled but has not yet engaged in much risk-taking behavior, let him or her know that your attention and help are available now without his having to resort to risk taking to express his feelings. If your teen's friends show evidence of such behavior, discuss ways one can say no and the importance of putting one's own safety and welfare first.

SET CLEAR LIMITS

Give your teenager a clear idea of what your rules, feelings and expectations are with regard to misuse of the family car, shoplifting and other risk-taking behavior. Be firm about what you will and will not tolerate.

Some preventive measures may be in order. For example, not all teenagers are emotionally mature enough to drive at sixteen. Emotional maturity, research has found, is far more important to driving safety than driver education. In states where taking a driver-education course enables a teenager to drive at sixteen, accidents and accident fatalities are higher than in states where teenagers can't be licensed until the age of seventeen or eighteen. If your teen is a very young and irresponsible or very depressed sixteen, postponing his or her driving privileges for another year or two or until she is more emotionally stable can be a lifesaver.

DON'T COVER UP FOR YOUR TEENAGER

If he is in trouble because of risk-taking behavior, be as loving and supportive as you can, but do not protect him from the consequences of these actions and thus deprive your child of a much-needed lesson. For example, don't try to pay off the store if your teen is caught shoplifting; if your child comes home with stolen goods, don't simply let him off the hook with a stern lecture.

Marilyn Peters recently confronted her thirteen-year-old daughter when it became obvious that the loot she brought back from an afternoon of shopping was stolen. "It was difficult to know what to do, but I called the store and told the manager that we would be in to see him," she says. "We went in and I made Jill give back the merchandise she had taken. I think she learned a valuable lesson. It was tough for me, too. I felt I had to show her how to do the right thing and yet tried to be supportive. I tried to communicate the idea to her that I loved her enough and cared enough to get tough and expose her to some discomfort to change her behavior."

If you continually shield your teen from the consequences of such actions, you are perpetuating the problem and keeping your child from learning and growing.

DISCUSS THE FEELINGS BEHIND RISK-TAKING BEHAVIOR AND YOUR OWN FEELINGS AS WELL

Express your concern over the teen's behavior and point out that it indicates underlying depression or other uncomfortable feelings, including low self-esteem (maybe your teen doesn't feel important enough to say no to friends who encourage him or her in risk-taking activities). Explore how the teen feels about herself and the world. If she is troubled, talk about things that might be changed for the better. Work on building your teen's self-esteem and confidence in her ability to cope. This will help her to make safer choices.

IF YOUR CHILD IS A CHRONIC RISK TAKER, SEEK PROFESSIONAL HELP

Risky actions are quite likely to be symptoms of serious underlying problems and troubling feelings. Individual *and* family counseling can be very constructive and may even save your child's life. Seeing risk-taking behavior as a sign of trouble, a cry for help, a misguided way of coping with problems and stresses is a vital first step in helping your child to grow and to change.

It is important that your child learn to grow past such behavior so that he or she will not avoid learning essential life skills and simply anesthetize her feelings with drugs, alcohol, sex and fast cars. Risk-taking behavior only postpones growth and complicates life. Teaching your child, by firm guidelines and by setting a good example yourself, that quick fixes and diversions are no substitute for the responsible, mature facing and solving of problems can make a lasting, positive difference in her life.

Part VIII

TEENAGERS AND SUICIDE

CHAPTER

26

Suicide: No Idle Threat

Shawn Stewart was seventeen, bright, handsome and talented. He was a model son in many ways, his parents agree. He had never given them a moment's worry except during those times when he became moody and withdrawn and locked himself in his room. Those moments, however, seemed insignificant in comparison to the good times—times when Shawn and his parents talked about his going to an Ivy League college and then on to medical school to prepare for a career as a surgeon. His life was full of promise and plans.

The depression that Shawn began to show that spring seemed completely incongruous with the realities of his life. His parents tried to cheer him up by pointing out how talented he was, how lucky he was, how proud he made them. But Shawn started withdrawing even more, spending hours alone in his room. He lost interest in hobbies and in school. When his grades began to slip a bit, his parents became truly worried. They were thinking about seeking help from a psychiatrist when, quite suddenly, Shawn seemed better. He was busy that Saturday, cleaning his room, writing letters and helping his dad in the yard. Nancy Stewart remembers that he seemed almost cheerful at dinner that night and recalls how happy and relieved she felt to see her son looking so much better. She had no way of knowing that only a few hours later Shawn would lock himself in his room, turn on the stereo full blast, take his father's handgun and shoot himself in the head.

The letters he had been writing that day pleaded with his parents not to blame themselves and told his friends which of his possessions they could have. Only in a letter to his older sister, who was away at college, did he reveal that he felt his parents valued him only when he achieved and his fears that they would not love him if they knew his secrets—one known, one suspected: He knew, without a doubt, that he was gay, and he suspected that despite his obvious intelligence and his good grades, he was not quite up to continuing his pattern of achievement at an Ivy League school and feared that he would never make it to medical school. While others saw his future as bright, Shawn saw it as hopeless and bleak, with parental rejection and disappointment on the horizon.

There are too many Shawn Stewarts—too many teens who feel hopeless and alone, too many teens who end their lives just as their young adult years are ready to unfold. The statistics are alarming:

- In 1990 an estimated one million U.S. high school students attempted suicide, and approximately 3.6 million students in grades nine through twelve (30 percent of all students in that age range) reported thinking of suicide during that year.
- The National Adolescent Student Health Survey in 1988 revealed that of the 11,000 teenagers polled, 25 percent of the males and 42 percent of the females said that they had given serious thought to suicide at some time in the past.
- About 5,000 young Americans between the ages of fifteen and twenty-four take their own lives each year.
- The Gallup Organization's National Teen Suicide Audit revealed that 60 percent of teenagers personally know other teens who have attempted suicide. Fifteen percent of those surveyed had considered suicide themselves. The study, the first documentation of teen views of suicide, found that 6 percent of American teenagers have attempted suicide.
- According to a 1991 report from the National Center for Health Statistics, 2,059 adolescents aged fifteen to nineteen and 243 young people under fifteen committed suicide in 1988.
- The rate of adolescent suicide has nearly tripled over the past three decades.
- Suicide is the third leading cause of death among teens in the fifteen-to-nineteen age range, with only accidents and homicides claiming more

young lives. Experts believe that many accidents are in fact thinly disguised suicides.

Who are these young people behind the statistics who try to take their own lives before those lives have really begun?

All types of teenagers commit suicide: those from impoverished homes and those from affluent ones, achievers and non-achievers, kids whose problems have been obvious for some time and those whose lives seem ideal. Suicidal feelings occur in many young people. "One study of college freshmen revealed that seventy percent had thought of suicide in one given year," says Dr. Lee Robbins Gardner. "So the adolescent who has such thoughts and is convinced that he or she is all alone should be reassured that these feelings are *not* all that uncommon."

However, adolescents who *act* on these feelings, who actually attempt or manage to commit suicide, tend to share certain characteristics, and they have been the subject of a number of studies.

• *Teens who commit suicide are most likely to be white males.* Teens most likely to complete suicides are white males; those most likely to attempt suicide are white females. While African-American and Latino adolescents have lower suicide rates, Native American teens have the highest suicide rate of the ethnic groups.

• *They are often seriously depressed.* The seriously depressed teen may have a sense of hopelessness: no hope for changing his or her life situation, no hope for the future. He or she may be too immobilized by depression to see any alternatives or to take any positive steps toward change. At the same time the teen who has been depressed and whose mood begins to improve can be a significant suicide risk. The reason: When the depression begins to lift—but before it lifts enough for the future to look hopeful—the teen may find the strength and motivation to act on suicidal feelings.

• *They have often experienced recent significant stress.* This may be the stress of a romantic breakup or academic disappointment. It may be an argument or continuing conflict with a parent or other family member or important friend.

It may be a real or perceived failure to live up to rigid expectations—either their own or those of their parents. They may be dealing with the stress of coping with a learning disability. Teens who have attention-deficit disorder have been found to be at particular risk for suicide.

• *They may be hostile, impulsive or delusional.* Sometimes a suicidal act is a way of saying "You'll be sorry" for the teen who is angry at parents or peers and who acts on impulse without considering that suicide is a permanent solution to a temporary problem.

Some teens delude themselves that death isn't permanent. Dr. J. Kronenberg and his colleagues at Shalvata Mental Health Center in Israel have identified "the Sleeping Beauty Delusion" as a particularly ominous suicide risk in adolescent girls. These girls, he found, display a common thought disorder that they might die by suicide now to be awakened or reborn via a kiss from a future Prince Charming. They fantasize reawakening to a better world.

• *They are likely to have a substance-abuse problem.* Drug or alcohol abuse quite often coexists with depression in teens; substance abuse alone can put a teen at risk for suicide. In a recent study, it was found that the *main* psychiatric diagnosis for 53 percent of 133 consecutive young suicides in the San Diego area was substance abuse. In half of these cases substance abuse was the only diagnosis.

A study at the University of Pittsburgh found that teens who commit suicide these days are ten times more likely to be drunk or high on drugs at the time than were their counterparts twenty years ago. And if intoxicated, the teens are seven times more likely to use more effective means—such as guns—and to succeed in their suicide attempt.

Dallas psychiatrist Dr. Frank Crumley, who has treated and studied a number of suicidal teenagers, notes that the most typical suicide candidate is a severely depressed, impulsive girl with a history of drug abuse. He found that these patients have a tendency to react severely to loss and to have poorly controlled rage. Most attempted to anesthetize their troubling feelings with alcohol or drugs and some 40 percent had tried to take their lives before.

• *They know someone who has committed suicide.* Teens with a parent or sibling who has committed suicide are more likely to do so themselves, according to a number of studies, among them a survey of the records of 6,000 hospitalized psychiatric patients. In this study, almost half of the 243 patients with a family history of suicide of a close relative had attempted suicide themselves.

In his study of teenagers who had attempted suicide, Dr. Alan Berman of the Washington Psychological Center observed that suicidal teens share a number of characteristics, one of the major ones being parents who had committed or attempted suicide. "The example of their parents may have taught the teen that if things get rough, suicide is a way out," he says. "Also, teens with a suicide in the family are often frightened that their own suicide may be predestined. They may also feel guilty about what they were not able to do for the deceased parent."

• *They come from troubled families in which communication is poor and dysfunctional boundary systems exist.* Several studies on families of teen suicide victims have shown that these families tend to show less affection and more hostility, with yelling and nagging the norm. A symbiotic relationship exists between parent and teen that allows no autonomy. The parents are either extremely lenient or authoritarian and may move often, which prevents the teen from establishing stable ties outside the family.

When families have dysfunctional boundary systems, the parents may lean too much emotionally on the adolescent, trying either to reverse the parent-child role or to replace a lost spouse relationship by casting the adolescent in the emotional role of spouse.

This was the case with Jessica, fifteen, whom I encountered several years ago in the studio audience of a television talk show in San Francisco. Jessica's mother, a drug addict, had deserted the family several years before, and Jessica was living with her father and two younger brothers. Jessica's father, who was a manager at the television station, had an active social life and relied on Jessica for everything: housework, care of the younger children, cooking and nurturing him (including listening to his dating problems). Jessica felt distinctly unnurtured herself and that "no one would listen to how I felt and that life would always be that way." She tried to commit suicide by taking an overdose of pills and had just been released from a psychiatric hospital after one month of treatment two days before this television show. Before the show her father bragged about how strong and adult Jessica was. Jessica was quiet then. But on the show she stood up to tell her story and began to cry, spilling her feelings about her loneliness, her myriad responsibilities, her anger that her father had no sense of her needs. After the show her somewhat shaken father asked for a counseling referral and promised to make an effort to be more sensitive to her needs and concerns.

Amy, thirteen, who split her time between her divorced mother and her remarried father, slashed her wrists after a particularly stressful weekend. Visiting her mother, she met her mother's new lover—a woman—who was openly demonstrative in front of her. Her mother told her that she felt she could be open with Amy about the fact that she was a lesbian because Amy was now "mature enough to understand." Fleeing back to her father's house, Amy got into an argument with her stepmother, who said, "If you don't like the way we do things here, go live with your mother!" Feeling hopeless and that she had no comfortable place to call home, Amy cut her wrists. She later told her doctor that she felt her parents were "throwing sex in my face before I even know who I am!" (In addition to the shock of learning about and meeting her mother's lesbian lover, Amy was adjusting to the birth of her stepbrother—her first sibling—four months before.)

Judy Winokur, a teacher at Amy's school, shakes her head when she talks about Amy. "This is one of those kids who is so accustomed to dealing with life alone that her depression was not easily apparent," she says. "Amy came to school every day and didn't seem particularly different during the time just before her suicide attempt. I did hear a lot of anger. We certainly have tried to be sensitive to what is happening with students, but we miss clues at times, too, if in fact these clues are ever given."

• *He or she has the feeling of being an "expendable child."* According to several studies, the concept of the "expendable child" means that there may be a parental wish, conscious or unconscious, spoken or unspoken, that the child hears or interprets as the parents' desire to get rid of him. The child feels that he is a burden to the family and that everyone would be better off without him.

"These young people have failed to win parental love," says Dr. Herbert Hendin, director of the Center for Psychosocial Studies at Franklin D. Roosevelt Medical Center in New York City. "Often the parents of a suicidal child want him around, but without an empathetic connection."

This lack of a warm connection can convince a depressed teenager that nobody cares, that life will never change and that only ending his life will stop the pain.

• *He or she may have a feeling of depression or hopelessness related to sexuality.* As we have seen earlier, gay and lesbian teens are at particular risk of suicide, quite often because they feel lonely, isolated and different because of their sexual orientation and because they fear or have experienced parental and/or peer humiliation or rejection.

The teen who has been sexually abused is at special risk, too, particularly if she takes the risk of revealing the abuse to a trusted adult and is not believed or helped.

• *The teenager is isolated without a network of supportive relationships.* This can be the teen who tends to be solitary and isolated by nature. In a five-year study of suicidal adolescents, Dr. Hendin noted that most had little emotional connection to others. "Those in college often used schoolwork to withdraw from others," he says. "Most of the college-age adolescents were unhappy with their lives but afraid of changes. However, the high school group engaged in a lot of provocative behavior and showed little interest in school."

Also at risk are those teens who are isolated from peers by family responsibilities and whose emotional connections are limited.

Eric, thirteen, was brought into a hospital emergency room after an almost successful attempt to hang himself. His suicidal behavior was triggered by a chance remark from his eight-year-old brother.

"This boy had a very sad and chaotic family history," says Dr. Charles Wibbelsman, who treated Eric in the emergency room and during his subsequent hospitalization. "He was the eldest of three brothers and only the youngest child, the eight-year-old, had an identifiable father, who was trying to get custody of the child. Eric adored his little brother and was functioning as the father in the family. He had an incredible amount of responsibility and a huge emotional investment in his siblings, especially the little one. Because of his many home responsibilities, Eric was isolated from his peers. His world was so limited and his focus so narrow that he was devastated when his little brother told him, 'I don't love you anymore! I'd rather live with my father!' His brother's rejection was the last straw for this already depressed teenager."

Many teens find themselves unable to break the cycle of isolation and hopelessness.

"What many suicidal young people have in common is the inability or lack of opportunity to express their unhappiness," says Dr. Michael Peck, a Los Angeles psychologist who has worked extensively with suicidal adolescents at the Los Angeles Suicide Prevention Center. "They find that their efforts to express their feelings of unhappiness, frustration and failure are totally unacceptable to their parents. Such feelings may be ignored or met by defensive hostility. This response often drives the child into further isolation, reinforced by the feeling that something is terribly wrong with him."

Suicide attempts reflect this feeling of helplessness and hopelessness. Yet many of these sad, depressed, desperate young people don't really want to die. They simply want life to be different. What a suicidal adolescent may actually be saying is "I want to escape my unhappiness."

It is crucial, then, to recognize the danger signs of possible suicidal behavior and to reach out to help before it's too late.

CHAPTER

27

How to Recognize the Warning Signs and Help a Suicidal Teen

The parents of Shawn Stewart and countless other suicidal teens were caught tragically unaware. That doesn't have to happen. Understanding the danger signs and symptoms of suicidal thoughts and behavior may enable you to intervene before tragedy strikes.

The Major Warning Signs of Suicide

- Severe depression or a sudden improvement in mood after a severe depression.
- A substance-abuse problem, especially if it is coupled with depression and feelings of hopelessness.
- Expressing feelings of hopelessness, helplessness and unhappiness and a general sense of futility.
- Giving away prized possessions.
- Withdrawing not only from family but also from friends.
- Talking about suicide or death as a release.
- Discussing methods of suicide or specific plans for a possible attempt on his own life.
- Previous suicide attempts.

How You Can Help

TAKE YOUR TEENAGER SERIOUSLY

Take *all* symptoms of depression, *all* comments about death, *all* suicide threats or attempts seriously. Don't dismiss such words or actions as attention-getting and manipulative. Don't assume that your child is bluffing about his suicidal intentions and urge him to go ahead. Don't lecture depressed adolescents, telling them how good they have it. That will only deepen guilt, depression and anger. See suicidal symptoms, threats and attempts as important messages from your child to you.

"You may feel that your teenager's suicide threats *are* manipulative, but that's not the real issue," says Dr. Alan Berman. "The real issue is that the kid is saying, 'Do something! I'm hurting!' If you don't attend to this, the fact that the behavior is manipulative may be academic."

Don't make assumptions that this, too, shall pass, that suicidal threats and fantasies will never be carried out, that the resilience of youth is ever present and will prevail. Instead, express your loving concern and willingness to listen.

SHOW THAT YOU CARE

This means taking the time and trouble to ask your child specifically about his or her feelings, even if this is a frightening prospect. Doing this will accomplish two important goals: It will demonstrate your commitment to help and, at the same time, give you some indication of your teenager's state of mind and the immediacy of the suicidal crisis. Some parents shy away, fearful that asking direct questions about depression and suicidal feelings will only encourage the teen to act on these feelings. Most experts contend, however, that this is not likely. Your teenager will be relieved that you notice how hopeless she is feeling, that you care and that you're willing to help.

How should you approach a young person who may be feeling suicidal?

"Try asking a number of gentle questions, each prompted by a yes answer to the one preceding it," says Dr. Richard Brown. The progression of questions that Dr. Brown suggests include:

> "It looks to me like you're feeling unhappy. Are you?"
> "Do you ever get the feeling that maybe life isn't worth living?"
> "Do you feel sometimes that you don't want to live anymore?"
> "What have you thought about doing to end your life?"

Specific plans for suicide are a sign that the teenager is in immediate danger. "If the young person has a method all thought out, she may require hospitalization," Dr. Brown says.

Unless you ask, you may miss this vital signal and the opportunity to help your child. You will also miss the opportunity to show your child that you care about what she is feeling and what happens to her. Asking takes courage on your part, since your child's distress is frightening and disheartening. You may feel like a failure as a parent because your teenager is so unhappy.

"Your child's depression doesn't mean that you're a failure," says Dr. Gabrielle Carlson. "Listening to her and helping her learn to deal with painful feelings is an important and maybe life-saving first-aid measure. After all, internal wounds are just as painful and in need of attention as external ones."

HELP YOUR CHILD RECAPTURE A GLIMMER OF HOPE

You can communicate hope by saying something like "I know you're hurting a lot right now and it probably seems that things will never get better. But depression, even serious depression, doesn't last forever, and I feel that together we can come up with ideas to change things for the better."

"There is one important fact that you must emphasize whenever you can," says Dr. Calvin Frederick. "That is the concept that while life exists, there's a chance that problems can be resolved. But death is final." Dr. Frederick also suggests that offering something tangible such as an immediate idea-and-feeling sharing session or an appointment with a mental-health professional will also give your teenager something to hang on to, a shred of hope that maybe life can change.

FIND SKILLED HELP

Professional help is vital when your teenager is feeling so depressed and hopeless that he is suicidal. This help may include crisis intervention and long-term counseling.

"Don't try to help by sheltering your child when he has a serious problem," says Dr. Lee Robbins Gardner. "Part of taking the problem seriously is discussing it with your child *and* with a trained professional."

In a suicidal crisis, suicide prevention centers, hot lines and other crisis-intervention centers can be extremely important and effective sources of immediate help.

"If your child hurts that much, it is better to take him to a professional specifically trained in dealing with suicidal crises instead of, say, starting with your family doctor," says Dr. Charles Wibbelsman. "Your doctor is likely to refer you to someone better trained for such a crisis, which wastes time and adds to the teen's anguish. He may feel: 'Nobody can help me. Nobody wants to help me. They keep passing me on to someone else. I'm going to stop trying. No one cares.' On the other hand, if your child's first contact is with someone skilled in suicide-crisis counseling, the immediate crisis will be dealt with sooner and more effectively, and if a referral for long-term counseling is needed later, it won't be seen in the same light—as a rejection in the midst of a crisis."

LIFE-SAVING CHANGES FOR YOUR CHILD MAY MEAN CHANGES FOR YOU

This could mean spending more time with your child or listening more empathetically or modifying your life in some way to accommodate change in your teenager's life. Such changes may be difficult and inconvenient, but they are crucial to your child's recovery from depression and, perhaps, to his or her life as well. Failure to see the value of certain changes and unwillingness to compromise will perpetuate the crisis or even mean tragedy.

"I'm afraid that this is the case with Eric, the boy who tried to hang himself because he felt rejected by his little brother," says Dr. Wibbelsman. "Eric's prognosis is quite guarded at this time. When he was hospitalized, he started getting counseling from one of the psychotherapists here. However, the last time I talked with Eric, he told me that his mother had angrily put a stop to the counseling sessions. The therapist had been encouraging the boy to live more of his own life, to be himself and become more assertive about expressing his own needs—in other words, to make changes in his life that would be advantageous to him. Such changes would shift the load of household responsibilities from Eric to his mother, and she would not stand for this. She accused the therapist of fostering insubordination and withdrew her son from therapy. Now life is back in its old groove for Eric and he is dangerously depressed. His mother just can't or won't realize the role she plays in her son's problems and how vital it is that there be some change, and thus some hope, in his life."

LEARN TO COPE CONSTRUCTIVELY WITH YOUR OWN FEELINGS

As the parent of a suicidal or suicidally inclined teenager, you are likely to be in a great deal of pain yourself. You may be feeling tremendous guilt and anxiety. Getting professional help yourself in order to deal with these feelings instead of being immobilized by them may enable you to help your teen more effectively.

The fact that your child is having a serious emotional crisis does not mean that you are a bad parent. The fact that you are aware and willing to admit that a problem exists and are concerned shows that you're a good and caring parent. You may need help in dealing with your feelings or in learning to communicate more effectively with your teenager, but the fact that you care enough to hear your child's cry for help, to face difficult facts about your child's feelings and your family life, to seek professional help and to make changes in your own life says a lot about you as a parent. None of this is easy or without considerable pain. So it's important during this difficult time to keep in mind that you have *not* failed your troubled teen. In fact, you may be playing a major part in saving his life by your listening, your love, your caring, your commitment to finding the best possible source of help and your continuing reassurances that as long as there is life, there is hope.

LET YOUR TEEN KNOW—AGAIN AND AGAIN— THAT YOUR LOVE IS UNCONDITIONAL

Often in adolescence and particularly in the middle of a crisis, expressions of love can get lost in the midst of angry arguments, hostile silences and uneasy compromises. Yet perhaps never will your words of love be so important.

An interesting thing happens in family counseling sessions when a therapist asks the parent and teen if they love each other. Slowly, hesitantly, most say yes. Asked to express that love directly to each other, the atmosphere of the room invariably changes dramatically. In place of angry shouts and accusations, there are whispers and tremulous reassurances and tears as the longings of parents and teens alike to reach back into the past and rediscover their love for each other begin to reemerge.

Whether said with words or with a warm hug, a listening ear or an outstretched hand, the sentiment "I love you not for what you do but for who you are: a unique, valuable, lovable person. We're in this together. You're never alone. My love is always with you" can mean a step back from isolation and hopelessness. It can reassure your teen that you care. Feeling that someone—especially a parent—understands and cares can change, even save, your child's life.

Part IX

REACHING OUT FOR HELP

28

How a Professional Can Help You

Help. Outside help. Professional help.

Help may be very much in your thoughts these days.

Maybe someone has said quite bluntly, "Your child needs professional help." Maybe you seek help in advice columns, magazine articles and books, including this one. Maybe you know another teenager or another family who is seeking or getting professional help and you're wondering if that might be the answer for your teenager's problems, too.

Or maybe you've reached the end of your rope, the limits of your resources to help your teenager. You feel frightened, guilty, desperate, angry and very much alone. You want to seek help but hesitate, unsure about what is available, affordable and best for you and your teenager. You wonder what professional help can do for you that you can't do for yourself.

Professional help can be found in a variety of settings and with a number of different types of mental-health professionals. While some people utilize such help to enhance already happy, viable relationships, hone communication skills and prevent major problems or crises from arising, many more seek help when a crisis occurs and they are not able to help themselves and their children. Whether professional help is utilized as a preventive measure or in a crisis situation, such therapy can help in a number of ways.

Therapy helps you to understand and come to terms with your own past. Our early expectations are very much a part of who we are. Parental voices—in the form of long-ago labels, admonitions, criticisms, predictions or praise—stay with us throughout our lives, influencing not only how we see ourselves, but also how we relate to others, including our children.

"Counseling helps you to understand your own growing up and what you may be projecting onto your child because of this," says Dr. Doris Lion. "Maybe you feel unloved because you didn't have rules in your home, for example, so now you have too many rules for your own child. Therapy can help you to grow up at last and find your own way."

With the help of a therapist, it is possible to discover and silence some hurtful voices from the past to learn new ways of seeing yourself and your alternatives, to develop new skills for loving both yourself and others and for living fully.

Therapy can help you and your family get feelings out into the open in a supportive atmosphere with a skilled professional who will help you deal with all your feelings in a constructive way. It offers relief from cyclical patterns of fighting, depression and hopelessness. "Therapy helps people to step back and give themselves a breathing spell," says Dr. Lee Robbins Gardner.

Therapy helps you to improve your communication skills, express feelings clearly and listen with new understanding to those you love.

Therapy can help your child find his feelings, begin to build a more positive self-image and make changes that will bring even more hope into his life, easing depression.

Family therapy can help mend hurtful patterns of interaction. It can help you break old habits that block communication, cause misunderstandings and perpetuate unhappiness.

Therapy can give you hope and direction in the midst of crisis. But professional help is no miracle, no instant panacea for all that ails you and your family. The possibilities mentioned above are the ideal results of professional therapy, not the inevitable outcome you can expect if you seek such help. How valuable therapy will be for you and your family depends on a number of factors, including how soon you seek such help, how carefully this help is chosen, your attitude about it, how you utilize the help (how hard you're willing to work, to compromise and to risk change) and how willing your teenager and other family members may be to do the same.

Do We Really Need Help?

The thought that you and your teenager might need professional help can be painful and confusing. It's hard to know where to begin, how to find the right kind of help. It's natural to have second thoughts or serious reservations about opening your heart to a stranger. And you may wonder if perhaps you're overreacting, if seeking professional help might be unnecessary. How do you know if you and/or your child need professional help?

Professional help may be in order if:

• You're caught in hurtful patterns of behavior that create and perpetuate problems and tensions.

• Your teenager is showing dangerous symptoms: an unrelenting depression that has gone on for more than a few weeks, perhaps with suicidal feelings; symptoms of an eating disorder; signs of substance abuse or another problem that has you feeling frightened and concerned.

• You feel that the situation with your teen is out of control and you don't know what to do.

• You feel depressed, depleted, angry, frightened or desperate about a situation you can't seem to change or have no energy left to change.

• Your family life is being seriously disrupted by your teenager's behavior or problems.

• You're finding it impossible or increasingly difficult to communicate with your teen.

• Your family physician, a teacher, clergyperson, school counselor or another professional in a position to evaluate your teen's behavior or state of mind has suggested that you consider professional help.

• *You* think that you, your teen or your family may need professional help.

Obstacles to Therapy

Even when you know, deep down, that you and/or your child need help from a mental-health professional, a variety of fears and feelings may hold you back for a time.

These obstacles fall into two general categories: emotional and financial.

The most common financial concern is, quite simply, "Therapy is *so* expensive! We can't afford it!"

It's true that therapy isn't cheap, but there *are* alternatives to paying from $50 to $100 and even $200 per session. A number of insurance plans and Employee Assistance Plans (EAPs) cover some amount of mental-health care—ranging from 90 percent to half or a portion of the cost up to a certain number of visits. Most community mental-health centers and family service agencies—as well as many individual therapists—offer sliding-scale fees that depend on one's ability to pay. A growing number of HMOs are offering psychological counseling on a short-term basis (usually about twenty sessions) with longer-term help available if necessary.

If cost is the primary factor keeping you from seeking help, check your insurance and HMO coverage carefully and look into community resources. Getting competent professional help early on can actually *save* money in the long run. If your teen can get help before his or her problems reach a crisis stage—possibly requiring hospitalization—treatment will be much less costly.

Some of the most common emotional obstacles to getting help from a mental-health professional are:

• *What will other people think?* Years ago a great stigma was attached to emotional problems, and seeking help from a mental-health professional was considered a shameful secret. While times have changed dramatically, traces of this mind-set may linger in some people's minds. Your teen, especially, may worry that his friends will think he's crazy if he goes to a "shrink." You may worry about what the neighbors or other family members or extended family may think about your going to therapy. But think about this: Why deny yourself or your teenager a valuable source of help because of the opinions of others? Have these others been able to help with your crisis? It's your decision, ultimately, whether or not to seek help *and* your decision whether or not to tell others about it. While there is certainly no shame in seeking professional help—indeed, it can be a sign of healthy, loving concern and commitment to change and to grow—your decision certainly can be private immediate-family business and off-limits to discussion with others if that makes you feel more comfortable.

• *It's too embarrassing, humiliating and difficult to talk about our private problems with a stranger!* It's not at all unusual to feel more than a little uneasy at the prospect of talking about intimate details of your life or painful aspects of your relationship with your teen with someone you barely know.

However, with the right therapist you will feel somewhat comfortable right away, and if you and/or your teen and therapist work well together, the therapist won't seem like a stranger for long. Your therapist has some unique advantages over your close friends and extended family: He or she is a trained professional and can bring a more objective perspective to the discussion of your problems. The therapist is there for only you and your teen during your scheduled session time and is bound by professional ethics to keep your sessions confidential. If you still find yourself having difficulty being honest with the therapist about family behavior patterns, secrets or conflicts that may be having an impact on your teen, consider this: There are times when helping your child must come before protecting your pride. Also, it's quite unlikely that you will shock the therapist. While each family is unique in many ways, human problems and feelings have many similarities.

• *I'm not even sure therapy works!* Maybe you have friends who have sought therapy with unanticipated results: Maybe they sought help for marital problems and ended up divorcing anyway; maybe a friend and her teen went for one session with a therapist and left disgusted and disappointed; maybe you've heard comments such as "shrinks are crazier than their clients" or have had a less than ideal experience with a therapist in the past.

While there are no guarantees that therapy is the ultimate answer to your problems, it may be time to give this alternative a fair chance.

What *is* successful psychotherapy? Being in therapy does not necessarily make everything better immediately. There may be very painful times as you begin to face feelings, issues and conflicts that have been obscured by problem behavior, denial or substance abuse. There may be unanticipated but not necessarily negative outcomes. For example, a couple divorcing after getting marriage counseling is not necessarily a living testimony of failed therapy. The therapy, in fact, may have smoothed the way toward a more amicable, albeit inevitable, parting.

While it's true that therapy doesn't always help, or help in the way you had hoped or expected, the outcome of therapy has much to do with the empathetic relationship between the individual or family and the therapist as well as the individual's or family's attitude, motivation and willingness to risk change. When these elements are missing, the outcome may indeed be disappointing.

But you and your teen can have a lot to do with the positive outcome of your therapy. The process begins with choosing the right therapist and continues with mutual respect, cooperation and hard work as you grow through your pain to positive changes.

29

What Kind of Help Is Available?

What comes immediately to mind when you think of psychotherapy?

Many people picture a dark office with the patient (or "client") reclining on a special couch and talking as the largely silent and impassive therapist listens. They may picture this scenario going on for years and adding up to thousands of dollars.

While some people still do undertake the long and expensive process of psychoanalysis (an intense form of individual psychotherapy with a psychiatrist or psychologist who has special training in the process of analysis) for a variety of problems, this isn't necessary or even desirable for many today. The trend these days seems to be toward shorter-term therapy in individual, group or family configurations. Whether the therapist is a psychiatrist, psychologist, marriage/family counselor, psychiatric social worker or psychiatric nurse, the process may last for a few weeks or a few months, with more serious problems taking longer to resolve.

Therapy can take a number of forms. There are differences in focus. *Psychodynamic therapy* focuses on talking: utilizing feelings, dreams and memories to bring up and resolve issues and conflicts that may be a part of your teen's depression and your family's difficulties. *Cognitive therapy* is based on the idea that people who are depressed or anxious have these feelings primarily because these emotional states are habits stemming from a distorted view of themselves. The focus is on changing this self-image in order to change the troubling feelings. *Behavior therapy* operates on the principle that certain behaviors, phobias and the like are "learned" behavior and can be unlearned via certain therapeutic techniques. Quite often, cognitive and behavioral therapies are used together and can be particularly effective in treating teenage depression.

There are also a number of different configurations that therapy can take. *Individual therapy* involves intensive work between an individual client and the therapist and includes current problems, past experiences, self-concept and other matters of importance to the individual. It is likely to be more present-oriented, shorter-term and more interactive than traditional psychoanalysis. *Family therapy* is devoted to treating the family as a system, focusing on the concept that most problems exist within the family system, not totally with an individual family member. Many therapists believe that a troubled teenager is often expressing symptoms of family conflicts through his depression or problem behavior. So one person may be the *identified* patient, but the whole family or significant parts of it may actually be treated.

In *group therapy,* a trained mental-health professional facilitates the discussion with a group of unrelated individuals who share feelings, experiences and observations in an effort to identify and resolve problems and conflicts. This can be quite helpful to teens who may share some of the same problems and feelings about being different and alone.

Crisis counseling, or *crisis intervention,* is emotional first aid to help an individual or family weather an immediate crisis, evaluate the situation and determine what additional long-term therapy may be needed. Such help is meant to be short-term, but can be invaluable in a crisis. Hot lines and crisis-intervention centers fall into this category. The helpers may be mental-health professionals or trained volunteers who work under the supervision of a professional. These helpers have been trained to listen and to help you sort through your alternatives and determine your best sources of further help.

Other sources of help include *self-help groups*—sometimes supervised by a mental-health professional but quite often made up of people with similar problems who get together to offer support and coping guidelines to each other. Some of these, including Alcoholics Anonymous, Overeaters Anonymous, Narcotics Anonymous, Al-Anon (for families of alcoholics) and Parents Anonymous (for parents who are having problems with their children), are based on Twelve-Step programs that enable some people—especially those with addiction or substance-abuse problems—to face the reality of their addictive or compulsive behaviors and find new resources to change.

Often an individual or family utilizes a variety of professional services—for example, individual and family therapy plus, quite possibly, a self-help group.

While these services can be found in a variety of settings, it can be particularly beneficial to your teen if a number of treatment options can be found in a single setting. In a recent UCLA study, researchers established pilot programs that moved mental-health professionals to primary care medical clinics where teens were being treated. The mental-health professionals worked as part of a team with doctors and nurses, providing short-term cognitive therapy and cognitive therapy and medication. This team approach was found to be most effective in helping depressed teens.

How do you know what kind of help may be best for your teen? That depends a great deal on your teen's age and the nature of his problems. Several recent studies have found that those in early and mid adolescence, essentially teens still living at home, do best with family therapy, while those in their late teens may prefer individual therapy.

"Generally in adolescence family therapy is the treatment of choice since most conflict centers in the family," says Dr. Donald McKnew. "If the teenager is extremely disturbed, he may also need individual counseling." Other mental-health professionals observe that teenagers also respond well to group therapy.

Who Are the Therapists?

There are a variety of mental-health professionals.

Psychiatrists are medical doctors (M.D.s) with specialized post-medical-school training in treating mental and emotional illness. They can treat people with mild to severe disorders, but are especially well equipped to treat those with severe disorders who may require medication. At the present time only psychiatrists, as mental doctors, can directly prescribe drugs such as antidepressants. However, many nonmedical mental-health professionals such as psychologists and marriage/family therapists have cooperative arrangements with psychiatrists to consult with and prescribe medication as needed for their clients.

Ideally a psychiatrist should be certified by the American Board of Psychiatry and Neurology, which means that he or she is a fully licensed doctor with special training in psychiatry and passing marks in a series of special examinations to determine competence in the field. (However, since this credential is a fairly new one, some excellent older psychiatrists may not be board-certified.)

A *psychologist* has a doctoral-level degree—a Ph.D., Psy.D. or Ed.D.—typically in clinical or counseling psychology. In order to be licensed as a psychologist, this professional must have completed four to six years of graduate study plus several more years of supervised clinical training and received passing marks on a special licensing examination in order to practice. A psychologist can be a good choice of treatment for emotional problems and disorders and tends to be experienced in testing and assessment, which can be useful when extensive testing is required, needed or suggested as part of the treatment approach.

A *licensed marriage/family therapist* (often called an MFT) has at least a master's degree in clinical or counseling psychology or in marriage/family therapy. This generally means two to three years of graduate level studies and, in most cases, a specified amount of supervised clinical experience before licensure. In California, for example, an MFT must have completed a master's degree plus 3,000 hours of supervised clinical experience with patients over a period of not less than two years and then must pass a difficult two-part licensing examination before he or she can practice independently. This type of therapist may do individual, couples or family therapy, working with children, adolescents or adults.

A *psychiatric social worker* (MSW or LCSW) has a master's degree in social work along with supervised clinical experience. He or she is especially trained to evaluate and work with emotional problems in a social context. Some psychiatric social workers have additional certification from the Academy of Certified Social Workers. This certification means that the degree is from an accredited social work program and that the social worker has completed the required supervised experience and passed a national qualifying examination. Social workers, like the previous mental-health professionals listed, must be licensed by the state.

A *psychiatric nurse* is a registered nurse who has at least a master's degree in mental-health nursing and supervised experience in working with emotionally distressed individuals. Psychiatric nurses may also be certified by the American Nurses' Association. Such certification means that the nurse has met degree and clinical-experience requirements and has passed a written examination.

A Note of Caution: Look for a therapist who falls into one of these professional categories, who is licensed (or eligible to be licensed) and who has a degree from an accredited program. Many well-trained, legitimate mental-health professionals call themselves "psychotherapists," but unlike the title "psychologist," this is not a legally protected designation. Theoretically, anyone can call himself or herself a "psychotherapist." There are, unfortunately, a number of untrained or poorly trained nonprofessionals who set up a shingle and call themselves "psychotherapists." There are also some equally poorly trained individuals who may call themselves "clinical hypnotherapists" and who may have completed only a weekend seminar in techniques of hypnotherapy, yet attempt to treat everything from weight problems to depression. While hypnotherapy can, in some instances, be a useful therapeutic tool, it is best used by a properly trained and experienced mental-health professional in the context of ongoing therapy. The bottom line: Look for a therapist who has a degree from a fully accredited school and who is properly licensed.

If you opt for low-cost therapy at a community clinic, your therapist might be a graduate student in training—someone doing a traineeship, practicum or internship—under the supervision of a licensed mental-health professional. Some of these newer therapists can do very fine work and are strictly supervised, and the cost of such therapy may be somewhat less than therapy with an established professional. It can be a reasonable, viable alternative if money is tight.

How Do We Find Help?

If your teen is in a suicidal crisis, call your local Suicide Prevention Center of Crisis hotline for instant help and later referral for longer-term therapy.

If your teen is depressed but not in a suicidal crisis, you have more time to look for a therapist.

There are many ways to find a competent therapist. You can get a referral from your physician, from local mental-health associations or local branches of national associations for mental-health professionals. These would include the American Psychiatric Association, the American Psychological Association, the American Association for Marriage and Family Therapists, the Academy of Certified Social Workers or the American Nurses' Association. You can also get referrals from the graduate psychology department of a local university or the nearest graduate professional school of psychology in your area.

A friend or relative who has had therapy may be able to recommend a mental-health professional or ask his or her therapist for an additional referral.

If you're looking for low-cost care through a community clinic, an HMO or an EAP program, you will be given a referral. But it's still your choice whether you think that you and/or your teen will work well with a particular therapist. If you feel uncomfortable with that therapist, you can ask for another referral.

Some people get discouraged if the therapist they first talk with—whether in a telephone conversation or in a first session—isn't a good match. They may decide on the spot that therapy isn't for them. In a sense, that's like saying "I read a book once and didn't like it, so I don't think I'll read any more books ever." Mental-health professionals come in many varieties and, despite having solid professional training in common, have as great a variation in personal style, outlook and personality as the general population. So there is quite probably a therapist in your area, a local clinic or your HMO who will be a good match for you, your teen or your family.

A Note of Caution: While many very ethical and competent therapists give free community lectures on topics of interest to parents and others, there are some who have specifically targeted lectures that are designed to recruit patients for a specific purpose. For example, some are "headhunters" for psychiatric hospitals, looking for adolescents to put into psychiatric units, sometimes whether they need it or not. Some even consult with school counselors or try to bribe school officials to get names or records of kids who may be having some problems. Fortunately, in the wake of widespread investigations and reforms these headhunters are less common these days, but it's best to be on guard if you go to such a lecture. A typical headhunter lecture might be for parents and would be advertised in local newspapers offering useful information and help for parents who are upset or distraught or don't know what to do with a rebellious, out-of-control or otherwise troubled teenager. When you go to the lecture, the headhunter will say something like, "Bring your teenager to me and I'll help you get back in control." This is music to the ears of anguished and desperate parents. But what it can mean is that, after a session or two, the headhunter will hospitalize the adolescent whether or not he or she needs it because the headhunter gets paid a handsome fee by a psychiatric hospital for each patient he or she admits.

As we will see in the next chapter, there can be many good reasons to hospitalize a seriously troubled adolescent. But hospitalization *isn't* invariably the answer. You need a therapist who can evaluate your teen with her individual best interests in mind.

The best therapist for you or your teenager may or may not be the one with the most impressive degrees and steep fees. What matters most is the therapist's empathy for your child (and for you and your family, if this is family therapy), a comfortable fit of personalities, his or her ability to help in your specific situation and his or her availability to you. (For example, if your concerns have not reached a crisis, being on a waiting list for a few weeks may not be a problem, but this is highly unsatisfactory in a crisis.)

Assuming a certain level of professional knowledge and competence and his or her ability to relate to your teen and/or to you and to work well together, your mutual respect and your feelings of trust are the most important indicators that you have found the right therapist.

Generally, you can tell fairly quickly whether or not you will be able to work well with a therapist. While most people feel a little uneasy at first, you will know, deep down, if not on the first meeting then certainly by the second or third, if you will be able to work with this person.

When talking with a prospective therapist, note not only whether or not this person has empathy and is someone with whom your teenager or your family seems comfortable, but also ask yourself the following questions:

- Does this person encourage us to work at seeking our own solutions?
- Does this person work with me or with us, helping us to develop new skills for communication, personal growth and constructive coping?
- Does this person listen well?
- Is this person conservative regarding promises of therapeutic outcome?

The latter is an especially important question. A good therapist knows that the outcome of therapy has many variables, including the motivation of the people involved to change and to grow. Given these and the unique nature of your own various personalities and relationships within the family, it's nearly impossible to make predictions in advance about how many sessions you'll need or the outcome. Beware of the therapist who promises to "cure" your teen in three sessions. Beware of the therapist who wants to take total charge and tell you precisely what to do. The object of therapy, after all, is to find your own way of dealing with conflicts and challenges. Change requires time, effort and commitment and is rarely easy or instantaneous.

A good therapist will be professional, caring, unintrusive and nonjudgmental. He or she doesn't take sides or assign blame. He or she will help a troubled teen to explore and to acknowledge flaws and problems in himself, his parents and the family. At the same time, a good therapist works toward helping to balance the teen's life view. This includes the task of helping the teen to see what's right about him or herself, parents, family and life in general. It is important that a therapist helps both the teen and his family to show each other mutual respect, in bad times as well as good, and to rediscover their loving connection with each other.

CHAPTER

30

Beyond Therapy: When Your Teen Needs Extra Help (Drugs and Hospitalization)

For some teens it may be necessary to use a combination of psychotherapy and drug therapy to treat their depression.

If your teenager is expressing suicidal feelings, especially if he or she has a planned method or time frame, your physician and/or therapist may be urging hospitalization.

Or maybe your teenager is so depressed that he or she just isn't responding well to psychotherapy alone and so the therapist suggests antidepressant medication as a useful adjunct to talk therapy and wants to refer your teen to a psychiatrist for an evaluation and medication prescription.

Drug Therapy

Despite your desire to get the best possible help for your teen, you may feel hesitant to take the next step. It was, after all, a major step to get counseling. But antidepressants? Hospitalization? It isn't an easy decision to make, even for the most well-informed parent.

There has been a great deal of controversy recently about adolescents taking antidepressants and becoming suicidal, as in the tragic case of Matt Miller, 13 at the time of his death in 1997. Matt hanged himself shortly after starting to take the antidepressant Zoloft. His parents filed an ultimately unsuccessful lawsuit against the drug's manufacturer, Pfizer, but have continued along with other activists to increase public awareness of the risks antidepressants can pose to teenagers.

Why some antidepressants appear to increase the risk of suicidal thoughts or actions in adolescents is not yet understood. Some mental-health professionals theorize that severely depressed, apathetic patients, when put on antidepressants, may regain a measure of energy and initiative, while continuing to be significantly depressed, and this makes acting on suicidal thoughts possible. This phenomenon is called rollback. Other professionals theorize that adolescents have different physiological reactions to these medications. Still others express caution in all ways—caution against believing everything one reads in the media and caution against unquestioning compliance with a doctor's recommendation.

Along with the risks, there are some very real benefits to teens taking antidepressants. Recent studies have found that the newer antidepressant medications, called selective serotonin reuptake inhibitors or SSRIs, especially when they are combined with cognitive-behavioral therapy, can be effective, short-term treatment for depressed adolescents. At present, only Prozac has been approved by the Federal Drug Administration for depressed children and teenagers. But doctors, not only child psychiatrists but also family physicians, have been prescribing other SSRIs such as Paxil, Zoloft, Lexapro and Celexa to adolescents.

Public alarm about the suicide risk among teens taking SSRIs has resulted in fewer prescriptions being written for depressed adolescents. Recent surveys show that, in 2004, the number of children and adolescents on antidepressants fell some twenty percent.

What facts should you consider when your teen's therapist or physician recommends antidepressant medication?

While fewer than 20 percent of the 4,000 adolescents who commit suicide every year are on antidepressants (and most teens who are taking antidepressants are doing so because they are significantly depressed and thus at higher risk of suicidal feelings or behavior than other adolescents), parents, quite understandably, are worried about what they're reading in the papers and hearing on the nightly news. This concern has been heightened by the recent decision of the Federal Drug Administration to put a "black box" warning—the most serious warning by the agency—on all antidepressant medication regarding the increased risk of suicidal thoughts in teens taking the medications.

Despite the concerns, there are times when antidepressant medication can make a life-saving difference for a depressed adolescent. "There are times when it just isn't possible to reach and treat a severely depressed person with words," says Dr. Donald McKnew. "I think it's malpractice to try talking alone with someone who is massively depressed. It can be an exercise in futility. Chemical treatment may get the person to the point where talking can be effective."

How can you safeguard your depressed teen when a doctor wants to prescribe an antidepressant?

Make sure that the prescribing doctor has knowledge about and experience in treating depressed adolescents. A doctor in any medical specialty can prescribe these medications, but it's best to have your teenager's medication monitored closely by a child psychiatrist or adolescent medicine specialist who is up to date on the latest information about teens and SSRIs and who will monitor your son or daughter closely. Especially in the beginning, before the impact of the medication on your teen is known, an appointment every four to six weeks is *not* enough. If a doctor is so busy that he or she can only see your child at long intervals, go elsewhere. If the doctor feels that medication alone is the answer, go elsewhere.

Discuss the advisability of low dosages with your teen's prescribing physician. This is usually the choice in prescribing medications. However, let the physician know that you prefer that your teen takes the lowest possible dosage initially until the impact of the medication—positive or negative— can be determined.

Know signs of trouble and watch closely for any troubling behavior after your teenager starts taking medication. You should be particularly vigilant in looking for expressed thoughts of suicide (either totally new or intensified after drug treatment starts), suicide threats or attempts, increased depression or anxiety, panic attacks, insomnia, agitation and restlessness, noticeably increased irritability, angry, violent behavior or aggressiveness, risk-taking, impulsive behavior, an extreme change in talking patterns (especially if your teen, quite uncharacteristically, starts talking a lot).

Enlist the aid of others in your teen's life to monitor his or her behavior in a concerned and loving way. This isn't about enlisting people to "spy" on your teen, but asking for help and input from teachers, school counselors, pastors or youth group leaders, extended family or friends . . . anyone who is in a position to observe any changes in your teen's behavior that could signal adverse reactions to medications.

Hospitalization

Hospitalization of troubled adolescents is another controversial option. Many teens do best when they stay within their own families to work out conflicts and issues as part of the healing process.

However, there are some instances in which hospitalization may be preferable, even crucial, for a time. Your teenager may need in-hospital treatment if:

- He or she has a serious problem with alcohol or drug abuse and needs a highly structured program in order to get sober. Those excruciating first days or weeks may be most productive when spent in a supportive, structured residential program. Sometimes these are hospital-based and sometimes these are independent facilities like residential drug treatment centers or a boarding school for troubled teens.
- She (or he) has an eating disorder such as anorexia nervosa or bulimia. These teens also need intensive, multidisciplinary care because of the complicated nature of their illness and also because they may need to get away from family dynamics that could be contributing to the eating disorder.
- He or she is suicidal and/or likely to hurt himself.

On the other hand, if a teen is simply somewhat depressed, rebellious, has difficulty getting along with some family members or has problems with school, hospitalization may not be the appropriate choice. Indeed, if your teen is feeling like the scapegoat for family problems or is having trouble keeping up in school, hospitalization might only make him feel more stigmatized or cause him to get further behind in school. Outpatient psychotherapy and, possibly, medication, can be helpful to a depressed teen. Problems with school might be addressed not only with family or individual counseling, but also with help from an educational therapist who specializes in learning disabilities and problematic behavior.

If hospitalization is recommended for your teen, be sure to ask the following questions:

- Why is psychiatric inpatient treatment being recommended and how will this help?
- What are the alternatives and how do they compare?
- What does the treatment program include?
- How will my child be able to keep up with schoolwork?
- What are the responsibilities of those on the treatment team?
- How long will my child be hospitalized?
- What are the costs? How do we pay? What will happen if we can no longer afford this treatment and, yet, inpatient treatment is still needed?
- How will we, as parents, be involved in the treatment, in the decision to discharge and in aftercare treatment?
- What kind of follow-up treatment is available?
- Is the hospital approved by the Joint Commission for the Accreditation of Healthcare Organizations (JCAHO) as a treatment facility for teenagers?
- Will our child be on a specialized unit or in a program accredited for treatment of children and adolescents?

In addition to hospitalization, some parents seek help from special schools or programs for troubled teens. There are some fine programs among these, but use caution when choosing one that is right for your child. Get recommendations regarding these from your physician or from the adolescent medicine unit of your local teaching hospital. Visit the facilities before sending your teen there. Talk with other parents whose teens have attended such schools and programs. Ask about the credentials of staff members: are most of the staff members' physicians, psychologists or licensed master's level psychotherapists such as LCSWs or MFTs? Beware of facilities utilizing primarily paraprofessional or unlicensed therapists or who have no supervising physician on the premises or readily available.

Making the decision to make use of psychotropic medications, hospitalization or treatment residency programs for your teen isn't easy. Unless your teen is in a suicidal crisis—at which point immediate hospitalization may be necessary—take time to ask questions and consider your options. These options may feel uncomfortable for you, certainly not what you ever imagined for yourself or your teen. However, it's important to keep an open mind when your teen is in crisis. Asking for and receiving special help isn't easy. But it can be life-saving.

31

Making the Best Use of Professional Help

How to Get Your Teenager Involved

Maybe you've found an excellent source of help for your troubled teenager, but there is just one problem: Your teenager stubbornly and angrily refuses to go for treatment.

Many teenagers are resistant to professional help, fearing that if they go to a "shrink," their friends will think they're crazy.

Other teens dig in their heels and refuse to go to therapy because it's a parental idea, while others feel unjustly accused of creating problems they believe are shared by the family.

Or your teen may just feel hopeless—certain that no therapist can possibly help or understand:

What do you do now?

If your teen is in grave danger from severe drug or alcohol addiction or is suicidally depressed, you may need to override his or her wishes and reservations, which may be clouded by chemicals or severe depression. Involuntary treatment, usually in a hospital, may be in order.

The solution is not as clear-cut in less extreme circumstances. If you try to force your moderately depressed teen into therapy, he may not be an ideal patient with an especially good prognosis.

What can you do to help him accept and make the best use of professional help?

TAKE HIM TO A PHYSICIAN FIRST

A physical examination can be useful in identifying possible physical contributing factors to your teen's distress. Also, your teen may feel less threatened with the prospect of going to a regular physician initially. If the need for ongoing therapy is indicated, he may hear this suggestion in a somewhat different spirit if it comes from a physician instead of a parent.

SHOW YOUR TEENAGER THAT YOU'RE WILLING TO PARTICIPATE AND RISK CHANGE

Many teens balk at therapy because they feel singled out, blamed and stigmatized, and they feel as if they are being hustled off to therapy to be "fixed" so they will be more acceptable to their parents.

If you show your teen that you see this as a family concern, that you want to be involved and to make changes yourself, your teen may prove much less resistant to treatment. If you approach therapy as "a way to help us all get along together better" instead of as "a way to straighten you out," you're much more likely to get your teen's cooperation in the process.

INSIST THAT YOUR TEEN AT LEAST TRY THERAPY

It's a risk, but one worth taking.

"You may have to get tough and make it clear how much you're willing to allow," says Dr. Judith Davenport. "Part of this tough approach is to say that things cannot and will not stay the same, that therapy is a must, not an option."

While some teens may dig in their heels further at such insistence, others may hear it as the caring message it is.

For a seventeen-year-old named Amanda, that message came through eventually. At first she went to therapy reluctantly, mostly "to show my parents what a dumb idea it was." Once she got to therapy, however, and saw that the psychologist was working with the family to facilitate change in the parents as well as the teenager, her attitude changed.

"I began to think, Well, if my parents could change a little, maybe I wouldn't mind putting out a little effort too," she says. "What a difference it has made! Insisting that we all go into therapy was one of the best and sanest things my parents have ever done!"

OFFER THERAPY AS AN OPPORTUNITY, NOT A PUNISHMENT

There is a big difference between presenting therapy as a necessity because a teen is so hopeless and presenting it as an opportunity for everyone in the family to learn something about each other and about communicating more effectively.

Viewing therapy as punishment will not only make your teenager feel angry, embarrassed and resentful about going, but if he does go, these feelings could interfere with the therapeutic process.

It is far more constructive to see and to present therapy as a great opportunity for growth: a chance for all of you to become a more loving family and to become happier, healthier individuals making a variety of life-enhancing changes.

GO YOURSELF AND GRADUALLY INVOLVE YOUR TEENAGER

You may seek therapy yourself and find it immensely helpful in dealing with your situation. In the course of your own therapy, you might involve your teen in small but important ways. For example, ask the teen to come in for one of your sessions in order to help you learn to cope or to communicate better. If the teen feels that you are the primary patient, she may feel less threatened by therapy. You can work out some conflicts in your relationship, and your adolescent may see the value in therapy.

If the teenager refuses to go to a mental-health professional even if her requested participation is minimal, try to get her involved in an even less threatening way. Dr. Merilee Oaks, for example, remembers seeing the mother of a very depressed fifteen-year-old girl. Dr. Oaks' only contact with the girl at first was by telephone.

"She steadfastly refused to come in to talk with me," says Dr. Oaks. "But the first breakthrough came when I called to talk with her mother and the girl got on the phone and started asking me questions like 'Why would kids go see a shrink anyway?' and 'Do people talk with you about things like sex and dope?' I assured her that they did, adding, 'Why not?' She replied, 'If I did that, you'd think I was *crazy*!'" After several phone conversations, the girl decided to give therapy a try, with excellent results.

Getting the Most Out of Professional Help

Many people seek professional help halfheartedly and are not surprised when miracles fail to happen. Typically they announce with an air of triumph that the therapy is not helpful at all and discontinue it after a few sessions. Others, in search of fast help or answers, become discouraged quickly when such instant results are not forthcoming and quit before the therapist has had the time and the opportunity to help them. Still others seek therapy yet sabotage all efforts to help them.

If you've reached the point of needing professional help, how can you and your teenager make the best use of it?

APPROACH THERAPY WITH REALISTIC EXPECTATIONS

Therapy is not a magic quick fix. It's hard work. It isn't just the work of the therapist, but a collaborative effort between therapist and patient or, in the case of family therapy, the therapist and the whole family.

"Many times parents go out in search of an answer," says school psychologist Sarah Napier. "They find some method of coping or communicating, try it for a week or two, and if it doesn't bring about change in that time, they say it's not good. Keep in mind that you've had these problems for some time and you're not going to change it all around in three weeks."

Change takes time and occurs most often in small, gradual steps rather than in dramatic breakthroughs. Instead of expecting total change within days or weeks of beginning treatment, make some realistic intermediate goals for yourself and your teen. For example, if you and your teen have found it impossible to say three words to each other without yelling, make some intermediate goals on the way to loving, caring and even enjoyable communication. Try to talk for two minutes without yelling at each other. Then try talking without yelling at all. In the interim you might explore what makes you both so angry and how to resolve these angry feelings in more satisfactory ways.

DON'T SABOTAGE THE THERAPY

You can sabotage your own therapy in a number of ways—by being dishonest with the therapist, by refusing to consider changes that might be advantageous to you and your teenager, by trying to entice your therapist into telling you that you are right and wonderful and that the problems lie elsewhere, like with your teenager. Keep in mind that you have plenty of friends who will give you that message for free. The therapist is there to help you or all of you find ways to work through your current problems, to build a new basis for caring and communicating.

You can sabotage your child's therapy, too, by refusing to become even minimally involved, by putting him or her down for needing help and by being too intrusive about the therapy or too quick to act if he or she expresses negative feelings about therapy.

Mental-health professionals report that they see examples of sabotage every day. "I'm seeing an extremely depressed sixteen-year-old girl now whose family is quite troubled," says Dr. Doris Lion. "If her parents would get therapy, too, her progress and prognosis would be so much better. Instead, they say, '*She* has problems. We don't,' and so the girl feels stigmatized. Seeing a child's problems as isolated is a trap. Generally, the family can *all* benefit from therapy, either separately or together."

Dr. Judith Davenport has some suggestions for parents whose teenagers are in therapy. "First, respect their privacy and don't insist on knowing all that goes on in the sessions," she says. "Let your child know that you're available to help, but learn to let go and let your teen be close to others. That is essential to growth. Don't put your kid down for needing help. I'm seeing a girl now whose mother tells her, 'If you were *really* mature, you'd be able to solve your own problems.' It takes a tremendous amount of strength and re-solve for that girl to get on the bus and keep coming to see me. And many troubled, depressed teenagers don't have that strength so they can't make the best of—or even get—therapy."

Don't be too quick to intervene on your child's behalf or to quit therapy if your child complains about it.

"When therapy gets tough—as it often does before things can change and improve—your teenager may try to pull you in to intervene for him," says Dr. Davenport. "Don't jump in to defend your teen or believe everything that he tells you at face value. Give the therapy and the therapist a chance."

If your teenager complains about the therapy, listen empathetically but remind him that change is often difficult and painful, that he may have to feel worse for a time before he begins to feel better. Of course, if you have serious questions about the therapist's competence or ethics, changing therapists may be in order. Usually, however, the best move is to offer your child en-couragement and support while insisting that he give therapy a fair chance.

KEEP AN OPEN MIND AND RISK CHANGE YOURSELF

In order for your teenager's problems to change, *you* may have to make some changes, too. You may need to change your communication style or to see your teenager's behavior from a new point of view. You may need to examine your own past, your attitudes and your relationship with your own parents and with your child. None of this is easy or without pain. But it's important to be open to the idea of making some constructive changes, if necessary, instead of expect-ing another person to do all the changing. Taking the risk of change—trying new ways of being, of sharing your feelings and of relating to your teen—is a way to get back in touch and eventually grow in mutual respect and rediscover your love for each other.

Such goals may seem distant right now as you and your teen struggle through myriad feelings: depression, anger, desperation and a great deal of shared pain. You wonder if you'll ever be close again, if you'll ever be happy again, if you'll ever have peace in your home again. No one can give you any 100 percent guaranteed promises and then make them come true instantly. No one can give you easy answers or guaranteed-to-work-in-every-instance suggestions for building a new relationship with your teen. But you need not struggle alone. There is expert and compassionate help available to enable you and your teenager to find new ways of reaching out to each other and of sharing all that life has to offer—love and anger, tears and laughter, growing pains and triumphs, bittersweet memories and brave new dreams.

Online Resource List

www.nimh.nih.gov
This is the website for the National Institute of Mental Health, a division of the National Institutes of Health. This site offers comprehensive, reliable information on depression, antidepressant medications, self-help and treatment options.

www.fda.gov/cder/drug
This Federal Drug Administration website gives the latest news about SSRI antidepressants and the black box warning regarding adolescents and suicidal ideation.

www.helpguide.org/mental/depression_teen.htm
This site offers information about teen depression, self-help, what parents can do and an in-depth discussion of treatment options. This website offers expert, noncommercial information on mental health and wellness in general. It is sponsored by the Rotary Club of Santa Monica, CA, as a public service.

www.nlm.nih.gov/medlineplus/ency/article/001518.htm
This site from the U.S. National Library of Medicine discusses teenage depression and its link with other disorders such as anxiety, along with signs, symptoms and useful tests.

www.about-teen-depression.com
Information about teen depression including treatment options and the ADHD/depression and obesity/depression links in adolescents.

www.psychologyinfo.com/depression/teen.htm
This is a helpful site for both teens and parents with information about symptoms of depression, types of depression, treatment, how to talk to others, alcohol and drug use and depression, suicide, and myths about depression.

www.focusas.com/Depression.html
This site from Focus Adolescent Services is an Internet clearinghouse that provides information on teen depression, a link to the FDA website for up-to-the-minute information on antidepressants and adolescents and a Directory of Family Help in the U.S. and Canada (featuring click-on programs, support groups, hotlines and helplines nationwide). A word of caution: therapeutic boarding schools and other residency programs are featured prominently in this mix. The quality of these varies greatly and this treatment option should be explored, ideally, only with the help and guidance of your child's physician or mental-health professional. If you are exploring such options online, beware of schools or programs not staffed by *licensed* mental-health professionals.

About the Author

Kathleen McCoy, Ph.D., is an award-winning author and psychotherapist. A former columnist for *Seventeen* magazine and a former editor of *TEEN,* she has written more than a dozen books and hundreds of articles for national magazines, newspapers and professional journals such as *Redbook, Reader's Digest, The New York Times, Family Circle, Woman's Day, Ladies Home Journal, Glamour, Mademoiselle, TV Guide* and *The Journal of Clinical Child Psychology.* Dr. McCoy has a busy private psychotherapy and life coaching practice in Santa Clarita, California, and is on the staff of UCLA Medical Center. She has made multiple appearances on *The Today Show* and *Oprah* as well as on *Home and Family, Sally Jessy Raphael, Geraldo* and *Hour Magazine.* She lives in Valencia, California.